More Praise for *Johns Hopkins Patients' Guide to Cancer in Older Adults*

"This clearly written book provides older cancer patients and their families with a useful guide to help them address their unique needs."

Michael Malone, MD
Professor of Internal Medicine
University of Wisconsin School of Medicine and Public Health
Medical Director, Aurora Senior Services and Aurora Visiting Nurse Association of Wisconsin

"Optimal cancer care—like care of other chronic illnesses—requires a partnership between the patient and his or her healthcare professionals. This partnership depends on a well-informed and engaged patient. The *Johns Hopkins Patients' Guide to Cancer in Older Adults* will prove itself indispensible in supporting patients and their families in this partnership."

Samuel C. Durso, MD, MBA
Mason F. Lord Professor
Director, Division of Geriatric Medicine and Gerontology
Johns Hopkins University School of Medicine

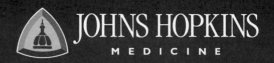

Patients' Guide to
Cancer in Older Adults

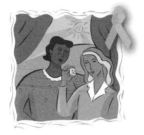

Gary R. Shapiro, MD
Chairman, Department of Oncology
Johns Hopkins Bayview Medical Center
Director, Johns Hopkins Geriatric Oncology Program
The Sidney Kimmel Comprehensive Cancer Center at Johns Hopkins
Baltimore, MD

Ilene S. Browner, MD
Instructor, Department of Oncology and Division of Geriatric Medicine and Gerontology
The Sidney Kimmel Comprehensive Cancer Center at Johns Hopkins
Johns Hopkins Bayview Medical Center
Baltimore, MD

SERIES EDITORS
Lillie D. Shockney, RN, BS, MAS
University Distinguished Service Associate Professor of Breast Cancer; Administrative Director of Breast Cancer; Associate Professor, Department of Surgery; Associate Professor, Department of Obstetrics and Gynecology, Johns Hopkins School of Medicine; Associate Professor, Johns Hopkins School of Nursing

Gary R. Shapiro, MD

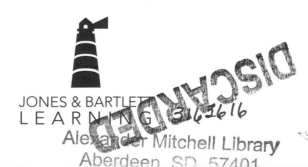

JONES & BARTLETT
L E A R N I N G

World Headquarters
Jones & Bartlett Learning
40 Tall Pine Drive
Sudbury, MA 01776
978-443-5000
info@jblearning.com
www.jblearning.com

Jones & Bartlett Learning
Canada
6339 Ormindale Way
Mississauga, Ontario L5V 1J2
Canada

Jones & Bartlett Learning
International
Barb House, Barb Mews
London W6 7PA
United Kingdom

Jones & Bartlett Learning books and products are available through most bookstores and online booksellers. To contact Jones & Bartlett Learning directly, call 800-832-0034, fax 978-443-8000, or visit our website, www.jblearning.com.

Substantial discounts on bulk quantities of Jones & Bartlett Learning publications are available to corporations, professional associations, and other qualified organizations. For details and specific discount information, contact the special sales department at Jones & Bartlett Learning via the above contact information or send an email to specialsales@jblearning.com.

The authors, editor, and publisher have made every effort to provide accurate information. However, they are not responsible for errors, omissions, or for any outcomes related to the use of the contents of this book and take no responsibility for the use of the products and procedures described. Treatments and side effects described in this book may not be applicable to all people; likewise, some people may require a dose or experience a side effect that is not described herein. Drugs and medical devices are discussed that may have limited availability controlled by the Food and Drug Administration (FDA) for use only in a research study or clinical trial. Research, clinical practice, and government regulations often change the accepted standard in this field. When consideration is being given to use of any drug in the clinical setting, the healthcare provider or reader is responsible for determining FDA status of the drug, reading the package insert, and reviewing prescribing information for the most up-to-date recommendations on dose, precautions, and contraindications, and determining the appropriate usage for the product. This is especially important in the case of drugs that are new or seldom used.

Production Credits
Executive Publisher: Christopher Davis
Editorial Assistant: Sara Cameron
Associate Production Editor: Laura Almozara
V.P., Manufacturing and Inventory Control: Therese Connell
Associate Marketing Manager: Katie Hennessy
Composition: Appingo
Cover Design: Kristin E. Parker
Cover Image: © ImageZoo/age fotostock
Printing and Binding: Malloy, Inc.
Cover Printing: Malloy, Inc.

Library of Congress Cataloging-in-Publication Data
Johns Hopkins patients' guide to cancer in older adults / [edited by] Gary R. Shapiro and Ilene S. Browner.
    p. cm. — (Johns Hopkins patients' guide to)
Includes bibliographical references and index.
ISBN-13: 978-0-7637-7429-5
ISBN-10: 0-7637-7429-4
    1. Cancer—Popular works. 2. Older people. I. Shapiro, Gary R. II. Browner, Ilene S. III. Title: Patients' guide to cancer in older adults.
    RC263.J59 2012
    616.99'4—dc22

                                              2010036986

6048

Printed in the United States of America
14 13 12 11 10   10 9 8 7 6 5 4 3 2 1

DEDICATION

This book is dedicated to our patients and their families, and in honor of our parents and teachers.

Contents

Contributors

Madelaine Binner, DNP, MBA, CRNP-BC
Nurse Practitioner, Medical Oncology
The Sidney Kimmel Comprehensive Cancer Center at
 Johns Hopkins
Johns Hopkins Bayview Medical Center

Grace A. Cordts, MD, MPH, MS
Medical Director of the Palliative Care Consult Service
Johns Hopkins Bayview Medical Center
Johns Hopkins University School of Medicine

Bryna Delman Ewachiw, PharmD
Oncology Pharmacy Coordinator
Johns Hopkins Bayview Medical Center

Catherine Klein, RN-BC, BSN, MBA, OCN
Nurse Coordinator, Geriatric Oncology Program
The Sidney Kimmel Comprehensive Cancer Center at
 Johns Hopkins
Johns Hopkins Bayview Medical Center

Swetha Manohar, RD, LDN
Clinical Dietitian
Johns Hopkins Bayview Medical Center

Leslie Piet, RN, MA, CCM
Advance Practice Case Manager
Johns Hopkins HealthCare LLC

Mya S. Thein, MD
Geriatric Oncology Research Fellow
Division of Geriatric Medicine and Gerontology
Johns Hopkins University School of Medicine

Richard D. Zorowitz, MD
Chairman and Associate Professor
Department of Physical Medicine and Rehabilitation
Johns Hopkins Bayview Medical Center
Johns Hopkins University School of Medicine

INTRODUCTION

How to Use This Book to Your Benefit

Older patients with cancer are unique, both in the problems they present with and the way their cancer behaves. The purpose of this book is to help you understand how cancer and age affect each other, so that you can make better treatment decisions for yourself or help an aging family member or friend do so.

This book is part of a series of *Johns Hopkins Cancer Patients' Guides* designed to educate newly diagnosed cancer patients about their diagnosis and the treatment that may lie ahead. The other books in the series are disease specific, with each book covering a specific type of cancer (breast, colon, lung, etc.). This book differs from the others in the series in that it focuses on a particular patient population (older adults) as opposed to a particular type of cancer. This book is intended to be used in conjunction with the Johns Hopkins Patients' Guide Book of the specific type of cancer that you have.

Many authors have contributed to this book; they reflect the importance of a multidisciplinary team approach to cancer care in older men and women. The medical team of the Johns Hopkins Medical Institutions and its Geriatric Oncology Program are dedicated to supporting older patients, their families, and friends who hear the words "you have cancer."

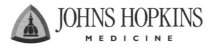

CHAPTER 1

An Overview of Cancer in the Elderly

By Gary R. Shapiro, MD

Cancer is a disease of aging. Contrary to what most people think, older people are more likely to develop and die from cancer than younger men and women. As we live longer, the number of men and women with cancer will increase dramatically. In the next 25 years, the number of people who are 65 years of age and older will double, and the largest increases in cancer incidence will occur in those older than 80 years of age.

Prejudice, misunderstanding, and limited access to clinical trials often prevent older patients from getting the timely and appropriate cancer treatment that they need. Older individuals may not have adequate screening for cancer, and when a cancer is found, it is often ignored or undertreated. As a result, older men and women may have much worse outcomes than younger patients. For example, older women with breast cancer have less breast-conserving surgery, less axillary node sampling, less radiation therapy, and less adjuvant chemotherapy. They do not always get appropriate adjuvant hormonal therapy, and their metastatic breast cancer is often left untreated.

Older adults with cancer often have other chronic health problems and may be taking multiple medications that can affect their cancer treatment plan. Because of this, they are often balancing on a tightrope, medically speaking, and it does not take much to push them off, be it the treatment or the effects of the cancer. Geriatric oncology addresses the special needs of the older cancer patient and their families who are concerned as much about overtreatment as they are undertreatment.

WHY IS THERE MORE CANCER IN OLDER PEOPLE?

The organs in our body are made up of cells, which divide and multiply as the body needs them, and cancer develops when cells in a part of the body grow out of control. The body has a number of ways of repairing damaged control mechanisms, but as we get older, these do not work as well. Although our healthier lifestyles have allowed us to avoid death from infection, heart attack, and stroke, we may now live long enough for a cancer to develop. People who live longer have increased exposure to cancer-causing agents (carcinogens) in the environment. Aging decreases the body's ability to protect us from these carcinogens and to repair cells that are damaged by these and other processes.

CANCER IS DIFFERENT IN OLDER PEOPLE

It is the stage-specific natural history of each cancer type that usually determines outcome, but age can alter the expected behaviors of some cancers. Indeed, the biology of many cancers is different in older people than in younger people.

BREAST CANCER

As women age, their breast tumors more frequently express hormone receptors (estrogen, progesterone), have lower rates of tumor cell growth, and have lower overexpression of HER2neu. The prognosis for patients with localized and regional stages of breast cancer with these characteristics is usually good. On the other hand, older women with metastases may have a more aggressive disease than their younger counterparts.

LUNG CANCER

Older people are more likely to present with potentially curable early stage lung cancers than their younger counterparts. Part of the reason for this trend is a change in lung cancer sub-types with age. There are twice as many squamous cell carcinomas in 80-year-old patients than in 40-year-old patients (with a proportionate decrease in adenocarcinomas and small cell lung cancers). Age may play more of a role in the course of small cell lung cancer than it does in non-small cell lung cancer; those younger than 65 do better than those older than 65.

HEAD AND NECK CANCER

Head and neck cancers are more common in men than in women, but among older patients, the percentage of women with these types of cancers increases. The known environmental risks factors (tobacco, alcohol, sun exposure, occupational inhalants, and human papillomavirus [HPV] and Epstein-Barr virus infections) for squamous cell cancers of the head and neck are not as common in older patients as they are in younger patients; indeed, advanced age itself may be one of the main contributing factors in the cancers' development. As in younger patients, head and neck cancers usually involve the larynx, oropharynx, or oral cavity. Elderly patients develop a more locally advanced (T4) disease, but fewer neck lymph node metastases. They are also more likely to have additional cancers (second primaries) outside the head and neck region.

ESOPHAGEAL CANCER

There are two types of esophageal cancer: squamous cell cancer and adenocarcinoma. The squamous cell type can occur anywhere in the esophagus and is related to smoking and drinking large quantities of alcohol. It is on the decline in younger people, but is still quite prevalent in older people who grew up in a less health-conscious era. Adenocarcinomas of the esophagus occur at the lowest end of the esophagus and are associated with gastroesophageal acid reflux disease. The overwhelming majority of the millions of people who have acid reflux do not get cancer, but those who have changes in the esophagus, a condition called Barrett's esophagus seen by endoscopy, have a much higher risk of cancer and have to be followed closely. Patients with Barrett's esophagus are followed by repeat endoscopy and biopsy. Since older people have more time for exposure to the cancer-causing effects of acid reflux, it is no surprise that the number of people with adenocarcinoma of the esophagus is increasing as people live longer.

GASTRIC (STOMACH) CANCER

Risk factors for stomach cancer include gastric polyps, pernicious anemia, prior *Helicobacter pylori* (the bacteria associated with peptic ulcers) infection, and prior stomach surgery (in which part of the stomach was removed). Stomach cancer is usually adenocarcinoma. There are two types of stomach adenocarcinoma. The intestinal variety of adenocarcinoma of the stomach arises in areas of the stomach affected by chronic atrophic gastritis, and since it takes years to develop, it is more common in the elderly. This type of stomach cancer has a localized growth pattern, and local resection of the tumor by endoscopy may be adequate treatment. The diffuse type of stomach adenocarcinoma occurs more often in women, tends to occur at younger age, and can spread through the stomach wall. This is often called "signet ring" type because of the appearance of some cancer cells under the microscope. Multiple areas of cancer in the stomach are more common in the elderly than in their younger counterparts.

BLADDER CANCER

Compared to younger patients, older people with bladder cancer are likely to have a more advanced stage invasive cancer. Tumor grade is also higher in older than younger individuals, even if the cancer is superficial. Indeed, advanced age itself may be one of the main contributing factors in bladder cancer development.

GYNECOLOGICAL CANCERS: OVARY, UTERUS, CERVIX

As women age, their tumors are more aggressive and resistant to chemotherapy. In those with a family history or genetic predisposition, ovarian cancer typically occurs at a younger age. However, in women with certain genetic predispositions, (specifically mutations in the BRCA gene), the risk of ovarian, fallopian tube, or peritoneal cancer can occur at any age, including over 70 years.

Most uterine cancers are *endometroid*. This type of uterine cancer is estrogen-related, and generally considered to be a low-grade, curable malignancy. Younger patients most commonly have this type of cancer, and present with early stage 1 disease. On the other hand, many older women have the *nonendometroid* type of uterine cancer. This is a more aggressive type of uterine cancer that often presents in an advanced stage, and unlike the endometroid type, is not related to hormonal factors.

As women age, there is an increased risk of in situ cervical cancer progressing to invasive cancer, and a lower rate of regression of cervical precancer. While older women are less likely to have active HPV (the virus that causes cervical cancer) infection than younger women, older women do appear to be at risk for a reactivation of a HPV infection from their younger years.

BRAIN TUMORS

Malignant gliomas, particularly glioblastoma multiforme, are the most common type of primary brain tumor in the elderly. Gliomas that appear before age 10 and after age 45 tend to be more aggressive and resistant to treatment than those that occur in other age groups. In seniors, even low-grade tumors are more aggressive than those seen in younger patients. Molecular biology studies indicate that there are specific age-related genetic alterations that determine both the clinical course of brain tumors, as well as their response to therapy. Advanced age itself may be a risk factor for developing brain cancer.

LYMPHOMA

Hodgkin's disease in older patients often has characteristics associated with a poorer prognosis: mixed cellularity histology, "B symptoms" (fever, weight loss, and night sweats), advanced stage, and Epstein-Barr virus-positive disease. Compared to younger patients, older people with either Hodgkin's or non-Hodgkin's lymphomas are more likely to have disease that is resistant to treatment. Indeed, age is one of the most important risk factors for lymphomas, as well as a key indicator of survival in the International Prognostic Index.

LEUKEMIA

Older patients with acute myeloid leukemia (AML) have a higher frequency of disease with genetic characteristics that are associated with resistance to treatment and poor outcomes. Preexisting myelodysplastic or myeloproliferative disorders are common in older patients, and AML that evolves from one of these is biologically more aggressive and resistant to treatment than other forms of AML. Indeed, older age itself is one of the most important poor prognosis factors, and a key indicator of survival in AML and chronic myelogenous leukemia (CML). On the other hand, older patients with chronic lymphocytic leukemia (CLL) tend to have less aggressive disease than those who develop it when they are younger.

TREATING CANCER IN THE ELDERLY

YOU NEED A TEAM

Cancer care changes rapidly, and it is hard for the generalist to keep up to date, so referral to a cancer specialist is essential. The needs of an older cancer patient often extend beyond the doctor's office and the traditional services provided by visiting nurses. These needs may include transportation, nutrition, emotional, financial, physical, or spiritual support. When an older person with cancer is the primary caregiver for a frail or ill spouse, grandchildren, or other family members, special attention is necessary to provide for their needs as well. Older cancer patients cared for in geriatric oncology programs benefit from multidisciplinary teams of oncologists, geriatricians, psychiatrists, pharmacists, physiatrists, social workers, nurses, clergy, and dieticians, all working together as a team to identify and manage the stressors that can limit effective cancer treatment.

Treating your cancer will also involve a multidisciplinary approach, using various techniques to target specific aspects of the disease. An overview of treatment options can be found in Chapter 4.

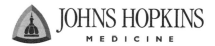

CHAPTER 2

JOHNS HOPKINS

M E D I C I N E

First Steps— I've Been Diagnosed with Cancer

By Catherine Klein, RN-BC, BSN, MBA, OCN

W hen you or a loved one has been diagnosed with cancer, the stress of trying to navigate your way through a complex healthcare system can be overwhelming. There is no convenient time to get this disease and the diagnosis alone can wreak havoc in a person's life. Getting organized early on is smart. Here are a few suggestions to help guide you through your journey.

LEARNING ABOUT YOUR DISEASE

You have just been told that you have cancer. You are bombarded with information from your doctors, the available popular and medical literature, and your friends and family. You might have difficulty absorbing, processing, and recalling the information provided to you. Comprehension, processing, and retention of this information may be difficult if you are feeling overwhelmed by your diagnosis or experiencing symptoms from your cancer or its treatment; this is often further compromised by the unfamiliar medical language used to describe your cancer and its treatment. The most powerful tool to guide you in your cancer journey is *knowledge*. Do not be afraid to ask questions. Knowledge can help you to gain control over your situation, and to make appropriate personal and medical decisions regarding your cancer care.

WHAT IS CANCER?

Cancer is not one disease, but a group of diseases characterized by the abnormal growth of cells that can result in the formation of lumps, masses, or tumors in any part of the body. Tumors can be harmless (benign) or harmful (malignant) to your body. Malignant tumors are cancer. Some cancers, like leukemia, do not form tumors; these cancers occur in the blood and blood-forming organs. The difference between cancerous and noncancerous conditions is that cancer can spread from where it started to different areas of the body, by direct extension to adjacent organs or through the blood stream or lymphatic system, in a process called metastasis. Even when cancer has spread to different parts of the body, it is still named for the place in the body where it started. For example, prostate cancer that has spread to the bone is called metastatic prostate cancer, not bone cancer.

TYPES OF CANCER

Different types of cancer grow at different rates and respond to different treatments. The cancer type refers to the organ or type of cell where the cancer started. Some major types of cancer include:

Carcinoma. Cancer that begins in the skin or in tissues that line or cover internal organs.

Leukemia. Cancer that starts in blood-forming tissue, such as the bone marrow, and causes large numbers of abnormal blood cells to be produced and enter the bloodstream.

Lymphoma. Cancer that starts in the immune system or lymphoid tissues. Tissues of your immune system include lymph nodes, tonsils, adenoids, spleen, thymus, and bone marrow.

Sarcoma. Cancer that grows from cells in connective or supportive tissue in the body, such as bone, cartilage, joints, muscle, fat, nerves, deep skin tissue, and blood vessels.

STAGING AND GRADING CANCER

The *stage* of your cancer measures the extent of your disease. Each stage may require a different treatment approach. To determine your exact stage, your doctor may order various procedures or tests to see if the cancer has spread to your lymph nodes or other parts of your body. These usually include imaging studies such as X-rays, computed axial tomography (CAT) scans, magnetic resonance imaging (MRI) scans, or positron emission tomography (PET) and bone scans. There are many staging systems, but the TNM system is the most common. This system provides you and your doctor with three vital pieces of information:

T: Size or direct extent of the primary tumor

N: Degree of spread to local or regional lymph nodes

M: Metastasis to other parts of the body

Numbers after the T, N, and M give more details about each of these factors. Once the T, N, and M descriptions have been established, they can be grouped into stages 0 through IV. Staging systems are specific for each cancer type, but generally speaking, the lower the stage, the better the prognosis.

> *Stage 0.* A precancerous state or carcinoma in situ. The cancer cells have not yet invaded into surrounding tissue.

> *Stage I.* A small cancer that is localized to one part of the body and has not spread.

> *Stage II.* A larger, locally advanced cancer that may or may not have spread to the lymph nodes.

> *Stage III.* A larger, locally or regionally advanced cancer that has usually spread to near-by lymph nodes, but not to distant sites.

> *Stage IV.* The cancer has spread beyond the region where it started, and has usually metastasized to distant tissues or organs.

You can have a clinical or pathological stage. A clinical stage is based on your imaging studies and a clinical examination performed by your healthcare provider. A pathological stage is based on an evaluation of your tumor and lymph nodes after they have been removed surgically.

In addition to determining the type and stage of your cancer, a pathologist will look at your biopsy or surgical specimen under a microscope to determine if you have a slow or fast-growing cancer. This is referred to as the *grade* of the cancer. The higher the grade of the tumor, the greater potential there is for aggressive behavior and early metastases. Grades are reported as 1, 2, or 3.

Grade 1. Slow growing or "well-differentiated" cells

Grade 2. Average growing or "moderately-differentiated" cells

Grade 3. Rapidly growing or "poorly-differentiated" cells

Do not be alarmed if the pathologist reports your tumor cells as Grade 3. This does not mean that you have an emergency on your hands, and it does not predict how well you will do. Grade is a relative term. Your tumor grade and stage will simply help your oncology provider to characterize your tumor and to develop an individualized and beneficial treatment plan for you.

FINDING QUALITY CARE

The task of selecting an oncology provider and a facility where you will receive your cancer care can seem like an insurmountable task in the setting of dealing with your newly-diagnosed cancer. Take some time to review, research and consider your options, but also be sure to ask your doctor how quickly you should take action. If you have not been referred to an oncologist, ask your primary care provider or specialist, or friends and family, for their recommendations. Consult cancer-based organizations and Web sites such as the American Cancer Society (ACS), the Leukemia & Lymphoma Society, the National Cancer Institute (NCI), or the Susan G. Komen Breast Cancer Foundation. Do not be afraid to ask for help in sorting through your questions and concerns and making important, life-saving decisions regarding who will treat you and where.

The Commission on Cancer, the NCI, and the National Comprehensive Cancer Network recognize and accredit hospitals and cancer programs that are committed to providing the best in cancer diagnosis and treatment and that offer a comprehensive approach to cancer care. The ACS, the American Society of Hematology, and the American Society of Clinical Oncology also provide information about cancer professionals, their backgrounds, and where they practice. Many cancer centers utilize a multispecialty team approach and offer a range of state of the art services in order to provide patients with the best treatment options available. Whether you receive your care at a comprehensive cancer center or at another institution or practice, you want your oncology team to be well informed about and experienced in the care of your type of cancer. They should also be sensitive to the special needs of older individuals with cancer. If you have a rare cancer, seeking your care at a comprehensive cancer center or institution where they specialize in your diagnosis may be beneficial.

You also may want to consider logistical issues when deciding where and with whom you will get your care for your cancer. You might want to consider the following: Does my primary care provider have privileges at the same hospital? How will I get to and from my appointments? Does the clinic have night and weekend hours? Does the practice have a consulting geriatrician or geriatric oncologist?

While thinking about where you want to get your care, you also should consider what you want and need in a doctor. Your relationship with your doctor is an important one that will probably last through treatment and into long-term follow up care. Some qualities you might want your doctor to have include:

- Experience with your type of cancer
- Experience with older cancer patients

- Board certification in oncology or hematology or other sub-specialty certification

- Affiliation with your health plan and/or accepts your health insurance

- Privileges at a hospital that is acceptable to you

- Factors that increase your level of comfort, such as languages spoken, gender, educational background, etc.

Many cancer centers have physician referral services available by phone or online. This service allows you to learn more details about the doctors in your area, such as their areas of expertise, medical certifications, languages spoken, etc. This information may help you to narrow your search. Once you have found a doctor that meets your needs, call his or her office and ask whether he or she is covered by your health plan and accepting new patients.

GERIATRIC ONCOLOGY PROGRAMS

Older adults with cancer often have different needs from younger adults. Older adults are more likely to have chronic illnesses, take numerous medications, experience social isolation, or have cognitive deficits. All of these conditions can affect life expectancy and the ability to handle stress, as well as the ability to tolerate, benefit from, and recover from cancer treatment. To address these differences, some cancer centers have developed Geriatric Oncology programs, which specialize in evaluating and treating cancer in older adults.

Geriatric Oncology programs employ a comprehensive approach to the diagnosis and treatment of your cancer. A multidisciplinary team works together to provide an evaluation of your health and functional fitness, as well as your ability to tolerate and benefit from the therapy needed to treat your cancer. The team includes your (medical, surgical, or radiation) oncologist and chemotherapy nurse, and also may include a geriatrician (a doctor that specializes in the care of older adults), pharmacist, social worker, nutritionist, psychologist, rehabilitation specialist, palliative care specialist, and pastoral and home care coordinators. Each program is different and each team is different. Together, your care team will assess multiple components of your global health and well-being. Such information can help your doctor and cancer team estimate how well you will respond to treatment and your likelihood of experiencing treatment-related side effects.

In addition to determining your cancer diagnosis and stage, a geriatric oncology evaluation will include a Comprehensive Geriatric Assessment (CGA):

- Comorbidities (other medical problems like diabetes, arthritis, and heart disease)

- Active symptoms associated with your cancer and your comorbid health problems

- Medications (prescribed and over-the-counter medications, vitamins, herbal, etc.)

- Nutritional status (changes in appetite, weight loss, diet)

- Emotional status (if you are experiencing grief, anxiety, depression)

- Social support (access to transportation, caregivers, finances)

- Cognitive function (your ability to think, reason, and recall facts)

- Physical function (performance of activities)

- Sensory function (vision and hearing)

- Gait (how you walk), balance, and strength

- Frailty (the ability to handle stress and stressors such as chemotherapy)

- Geriatric syndromes (for example, falls, dementia, and your ability to control bowel or bladder function)

Your treatment plan will be based on your personal and treatment goals and wishes, your tumor type and disease stage, and your physiological age (*not* your chronological age), as determined by your CGA.

If you are 80 years of age or older, or if you are older than 65 years and have other active health issues besides your cancer, a geriatric oncology program may be beneficial in helping you to receive highly individualized cancer care.

YOUR FIRST APPOINTMENT

To receive the best care possible, it is important for you to prepare for your appointment in advance. Sometimes it is hard to remember complex medical information when you are anxious or nervous, so ask a friend or a family member to accompany you to your appointment and to take notes during the visit. Prior to your appointment, make a list of any questions you have about your cancer, treatment, or other health concerns; this list will help you remember what you want to discuss with your provider. You should also make a list of the medicines you are currently taking, including any over-the-counter medicines, vitamins, or nutritional or herbal supplements. If you are on numerous medications, you should bring them with you to your appointment. If you have had any studies or procedures performed at a different facility from the one where your cancer provider practices, remember to bring copies of any reports and the actual films or a burned CD of any imaging studies.

When you meet your provider for the first time, you might want to ask some of the following questions:

- What is my diagnosis?

- What is my cancer's stage?

- Do I need any more tests or procedures before beginning treatment?

- What do my biopsy (pathology) results mean?

- What impact will the cancer have on my life expectancy?

- What are the goals of treatment: cure or palliation?

- What treatment(s) are recommended for my cancer? Why?

- When should I begin treatment?

- What are the risks and side effects of my treatment?

- How long will treatment last?

- Am I too frail for treatment? How is this decided?

- Are there other treatments available?

- What are my oncology provider's office hours?

- How can I reach a provider after hours?

- Who else will be on my healthcare team?

- Who do I call if I need prescription refills?

- Who do I call if you have questions about appointments, test results, etc.?

Do not be afraid to ask questions. Many patients have difficulty understanding the complicated medical terminology used to discuss their cancer and its treatment. Do not assume that your provider or your friends and family will recognize when you do not understand what has just been said. If you feel overwhelmed by the amount of information or you do not understand something said by your provider, say so. If you want more information about your cancer or treatment, ask your provider to suggest some reading materials or other educational resources.

During your first visit, you also should ask about the process for scheduling follow-up appointments, getting test results, and getting prescriptions filled. Your provider may have designated people in the office to handle these tasks; if so, ask for their names and contact information. Also, obtain a telephone number to call for help 24 hours a day, 7 days a week. The person you talk to during "off hours" may not be your regular oncology provider, so be prepared to provide some information about your diagnosis, your treatment, and any medicines you are taking. In order to be prepared in an emergency, consider keeping an index card with all of your pertinent information—your cancer diagnosis, other health problems, medications, current treatment, and date of last treatment—near your phone and in your wallet. Be sure to update it periodically to reflect any changes in your care.

GATHERING RECORDS

As you begin your cancer journey, it is important to keep your medical information well organized and to obtain copies of all of your pertinent data. First, request a copy of the pathologist's biopsy summary report. You also may need to obtain your pathology slides if you are seeking treatment at a different facility from where the biopsy was obtained, or if you are seeking a second opinion consultation. An accredited cancer center is required to review the pathology slides to verify their accuracy; occasionally, a review of your slides by a pathologist that specializes in your disease may reveal that the pathology or staging is different from the initial report. This review could possibly change your provider's recommendations for your cancer treatment. Accuracy is critical! Your treatment plan at every step is based on this initial information being correct.

As you meet with the different providers of your healthcare team, you will most likely gather large amounts of paperwork, test results, and personal notes. Create a system for all of these papers, as a good system will allow you to make the most of your time with your healthcare providers by having your information readily available and close at hand. The easiest way to obtain your records is to ask for a copy of your test results when you review them with your doctor or nurse. Getting records later is possible, but it might be harder and copy fees can be high. If you have your labs drawn or imaging studies performed at an outside facility, remember to ask them to send a copy of the results to your cancer care provider. No matter who sees you—a surgeon, medical oncologist, or radiation oncologist—they will want to review your imaging studies, so remember to request a copy of the actual films or a CD copy of your imaging studies (such as CAT scans or MRIs).

GETTING A SECOND OPINION

It is not unusual for a patient to get a second opinion after an initial consultation. A second opinion does not mean that you are unhappy with your doctor or that you plan to change doctors. It is not pushy or offensive to your doctor if you want to get a second opinion. You should not rush important decisions about your health, and a second opinion may provide you with additional information about your cancer diagnosis and another perspective on treatment options. Getting a second opinion also may help reassure you that you are choosing the most appropriate therapy, provided by a team with whom you feel comfortable and trust.

Your doctor also may get a second opinion for you by presenting your case to a multidisciplinary tumor board for evaluation of your diagnosis and treatment plan. Many cancer centers have tumor boards in which the patient's history, pathology slides, and imaging studies are presented to a team of providers from several cancer disciplines. They discuss the case and make treatment recommendations. Geriatric oncology programs also utilize a multidisciplinary approach. These programs have patient management conferences in which a panel of professionals discuss cases and make suggestions regarding patient care *during* cancer treatment. Multidisciplinary evaluations have the advantage of getting more than one doctors' opinion and addressing more than just your cancer.

YOUR CANCER CARE TEAM

Cancer treatment can be complex. It is not uncommon to have a number of different oncology professionals on your care team to help you throughout your cancer journey. Your team will help you to develop a comprehensive treatment plan according to your goals, specific diagnosis, medical condition(s), and overall health status. The members of your medical team vary from patient to patient, but your cancer care team members may include:

- *Surgical oncologist.* A surgeon who specializes in cancer surgery and the diagnosis and treatment of surgical patients with cancer. A surgical oncologist may be a general surgical oncologist, or they may specialize in a particular area of the body or type of cancer. A surgical oncologist may be the first doctor that you will see.

- *Medical oncologist.* A physician who specializes in systemic treatments for cancer. They treat patients using chemotherapy, hormonal therapy, immunotherapy, or targeted therapy. They may be a general medical oncologist or specialize in a particular cancer type. Consultation with this doctor is usually scheduled after your diagnosis is confirmed by biopsy or a few weeks after your initial surgery.

- *Geriatric oncologist.* A medical oncologist who specializes in the care of older adults with cancer.

- *Radiation oncologist.* A physician who specializes in radiation treatments for cancer, using an energy called ionizing radiation to kill cancer cells. Radiation therapy is often used in combination with surgery, chemotherapy, and hormonal therapy to treat many types of cancer.

- *Primary care provider.* This is the healthcare provider who you see regularly for ongoing care of your chronic and acute health needs. He or she probably knows you better than any of the other members of your cancer care team, and can be a valuable partner and resource for your new cancer specialists.

- *Pathologist.* One of the most important people on your team, although you will probably never meet this person. Your pathologist looks at your tissue under a microscope to determine the type and size of your tumor, as well as provides other prognostic information that is used to determine your treatment plan.

- *Nurses.* You may meet surgical nurses, oncology nurses, radiation therapy nurses, and research nurses. Nurses will have a very important role in your care. Nurses will provide you with education, assess your clinical needs, administer chemotherapy drugs, and help you with physical and emotional issues.

- *Nurse practitioner (NP).* NPs are advanced practice nurses who are educated in a particular field of practice. They can help you in many of the same ways that your doctors do. Your NP will help you to manage your symptoms, care for you during treatment, write your prescriptions, and order lab tests.

- *Physician assistant (PA).* PAs help doctors care for you in the same manner as NPs. They may be involved in your diagnosis and treatment, as well as during follow-up visits after your treatment.

Other members of your team might include:

- *Social worker.* A social worker can help you and your family cope with the changes and stresses that often occur with a diagnosis of cancer. Social workers can identify local resources for patients such as lodging, transportation, financial and community support resources, and home healthcare and hospice services.

- *Dietician.* Cancer patients often have special dietary needs because of the effects of their cancer and its therapy. A dietician may advise you on how to manage problems such as loss of appetite, changes in your sense of taste, nausea, vomiting, or weight loss.

- *Palliative care specialist.* A physician or care provider that specializes in symptom management and in end-of-life care.

- *Mental health specialists.* The stress of dealing with cancer can impact your emotional and physical well-being. Psychiatrists, psychologists, social workers, and counselors can talk with you to evaluate your concerns and make recommendations or provide treatment to improve your emotional well-being. Anxiety and depression are examples of some of the emotional difficulties they can help with.

- *Pharmacist.* Pharmacists are trained to prepare and distribute medicines and to give information about them. Oncology pharmacists have special training in how to design, give, monitor, and change chemotherapy for cancer patients. They are familiar with medication ingredients, interactions, cautions, and hints for managing side effects.

- *Physical therapists.* Your physician may recommend that you meet with a physical therapist to help restore or improve your strength, flexibility, and stamina. A physical therapist can develop a treatment plan uniquely tailored to your physical needs, including exercise, massage, and heat and cold applications.

- *Occupational therapists.* Some patients find that they need help with performing certain skills and movements that are necessary for daily activities, for things such as personal care, childcare, or work duties. Based on a person's individual needs, an occupational therapist can offer patients special training using adaptive aids or methods to complete specific tasks safely and efficiently.

- *Chaplain.* Many patients find strength and comfort in the practice of their faith, whether through prayer, meditation, religious counsel, worship, or other rituals. The chaplain's job is to help patients and their caregivers negotiate their own path, no matter where it leads.

- *YOU!* You are at the core of your cancer care team. Never forget that *you* have the final voice in making decisions regarding what happens to you.

NAVIGATION SERVICES

Since cancer care can be complex, a growing number of cancer centers offer patient navigator services to help guide you through the healthcare system and your cancer care. A navigator may be a nurse, social worker, or case manager. When you schedule your first appointment, you might want to inquire about the availability of this service.

A patient navigator can:

- Help coordinate your multifaceted care with all of your healthcare providers

- Help you get your questions answered

- Direct you to local resources and support services

- Help you keep track of and find ways to get to your appointments

- Help you address personal issues that arise during your treatment

- Help you fill out insurance forms

- Help you find ways to pay for health care if you do not have insurance

UNDERSTANDING YOUR HEALTHCARE COVERAGE

Cancer care is complicated and expensive. Whether your medical insurance is from a private source or is government-funded, you need to investigate what your plan will cover prior to starting your treatment. You also will need to reassess your coverage as you transition through different aspects of your cancer care. Important information about your insurance coverage includes:

- What are the limitations of your policy?

- What are you expected to pay out of your own pocket?

- What services, procedures, and treatments will your policy cover?

- Is there a limit to how much your insurance will cover for treatment?

- Where can you get your care?

- Do you have prescription drug coverage, and if so, what does it cover?

- Do you qualify for any assistance programs?

- What is the authorization and certification process?

- Are case managers available to assist you with any insurance-based issues?

- Is there someone in your oncology provider's office who can help answer questions about your health insurance coverage and medical bills?

If you do not have medical insurance, or if you have limited coverage, do not get discouraged. Contact your cancer center and ask to speak with a social worker. The social worker may be able to identify resources available for patients who meet financial (and other) criteria for help in covering your cancer-related treatment expenses, including prescription drug coverage. The social worker may be able to assist you with nontreatment-related expenses as well, such as transportation and food costs. The social worker also can assist you in gathering any needed information and in completing any required forms.

Not all cancer care providers accept all insurance plans. Going "out of network" can leave you with large out-of-pocket expenses. Check with your provider's office to find out whether he or she accepts your insurance. Find out where you can go to get your blood drawn and imaging studies performed. You may be able to get your blood drawn at your oncologist's office, but it may be less expensive to have it drawn at a separate laboratory. When planning your budget, it is important to determine upfront what your insurance will pay towards medical costs. Many cancer centers have financial assistants available to help you understand the coverage provided by your plan, and many insurance companies provide you with a case manager at no cost. Case managers also can help you to navigate through your insurance coverage and how it applies to your cancer care.

Your insurance company may require referrals for particular aspects of your care. Referrals are often needed in order to see certain specialists, get selected tests done, have surgery authorized, and obtain other treatments. Claims may be denied if a referral is not obtained in advance. When you schedule any medical appointments, be sure to ask if a referral is needed.

You may be offered enrollment in a clinical trial. Some or all aspects may or may not be covered under your insurance plan. If participating in a clinical trial, a research coordinator or nurse will review your eligibility and insurance coverage prior to initiating treatment. Be sure to ask questions about your coverage of trial-based procedures and therapy prior to beginning your treatment.

TRANSPORTATION

Getting to and from medical appointments can be challenging and expensive, especially if you do not or cannot (because of illness or fatigue) drive. Some cancer centers have a dedicated transportation coordinator. If you need help with transportation, here are some suggestions:

- The ACS' *Road to Recovery* program is available in some areas. This program is made up of volunteers who help drive patients to hospitals and clinics for treatment. The ACS also may provide some help with the cost of gas. Contact your local ACS for more information about the programs available in your area.

- County departments of social services provide travel assistance for people who qualify. This may take the form of payment or reimbursement for gas, reduced fares for public transportation, or using a van pool.

- Many community and religious groups provide assistance with travel, or its costs, for people in their area.

If you need help locating services within your community, contact the cancer center and ask to speak to your patient navigator or a social worker.

CAREGIVER ISSUES

You are not alone! In many cases, it takes a village to treat cancer and care for the patient physically, emotionally, and spiritually. Cancer not only affects the patient, but also the patient's family and friends. Your caregivers and supports share in your successes and your stress.

As people live longer, have smaller families, and move away from home, caregiver issues can become more difficult. In the past, extended families and children took care of their aged parents and relatives. In today's world, families are sometimes living in several different states and there may be only one or no family members in the same city or state as the patient. Helping to care for a friend or family member locally or from a distance can be a challenge. Caregiver duties include coordinating the myriad of appointments; managing the routine day-to-day needs of the patient; meeting transportation and safety needs; serving as a liaison among family, friends, and multiple personal and medical caregivers; providing emotional, physical, and sometimes financial support; and juggling the demands of their own health, work, and family. After being diagnosed with cancer, a person typically needs additional help in dealing with their cancer and other health problems. An older person with cancer may have even more needs, and an elderly caregiver caring for a sick friend or relative is at significant risk of becoming overwhelmed and ill themselves if they do not have additional support from family and friends, healthcare providers, and their community. The tasks can seem insurmountable.

To help balance the needs of the patient with the well-being of the caregiver, consider having someone act as the point person and be in charge of maintaining a calendar of medical appointments. This person also should keep all parties informed with either Internet communications or conference calls when possible. Work with the strengths and availability of those willing to help with the care of your family member or friend. Family and friends who do not live nearby could contribute by doing things like sending cards, making frequent telephone calls, or researching resources available to the local caregiver. There also should be alternate caregivers available to give respite care when needed by the primary caregiver. Without adequate respite, the primary caregiver is also at risk for health problems, stress, and burnout. If your caregivers do not take care of themselves, they will not be able to help you. See Chapter 12 for information about resources for caregivers.

FAMILY MEDICAL LEAVE ACT

Serving as a caregiver can be both rewarding and stressful. Taking time off from work to care for a sick relative or accompany them to appointments can present financial and logistical hardships for some family members, but it has to be done, as skipping appointments or not going to the doctor may result in a visit to the emergency room and a stay in the hospital.

Check with your employer or human resources department to see if you or your family members qualify for benefits under the Family Medical Leave Act (FMLA). Those who qualify for FMLA can take up to twelve weeks of unpaid leave per year to take care of a sick relative. Get the FMLA paperwork signed by one of your relative's doctors. Some work places have you use your sick and vacation time first while others simply allow the unpaid leave. The FMLA helps protect your job if you have to take multiple days off to help care for your relative. You can find additional information about FMLA at the United States Department of Labor (866-4-USA-DOL [487-2365] or http://www.dol.gov).

COMMUNITY SERVICES

Community services are a valuable adjunct to the care that you can provide as a primary caregiver. You may want to contact either your local office on aging or a social worker to get further information on available services. Some services may be free or covered by your insurance, and others may have an associated cost (e.g., home health aides, sitters, and house cleaning services). You also may want to contact your place of worship or local organizations, such as the Veterans of Foreign Wars (VFW) post, for assistance.

An organization like Meals on Wheels may be able to help with making sure that an older patient has hot meals, with the added bonus of an expected visitor!

Case management may be available through some insurance groups. Consider calling the customer service phone number on your insurance card and asking if you have access to a case manager. A nurse or a social worker may be assigned to your case and would be available to help you to understand insurance benefits, to navigate the healthcare system, and to access community services. A case manager may save you time and energy that you would spend on figuring out how to obtain services you may need. If you have the financial means, you may also consider hiring a private case manager. The Web site http://www.caremanager.org has a dedicated section on locating a geriatric case manager.

CHAPTER 3

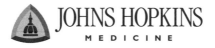

DECISION MAKING: SEVEN PRACTICAL STEPS

BY GARY R. SHAPIRO, MD

---

1. GET A DIAGNOSIS

No matter how typical the signs and symptoms, first impressions are sometimes wrong. Although most breast and lung masses in older people are malignant, some are benign or one of the slower growing types of breast or lung cancer that can be easily cured. That suspicious mass in your pancreas may not be a carcinoma, but an endocrine tumor that, though malignant, requires relatively simple treatment. Enlarged lymph nodes may be a sign of lymphoma, but other types of cancer often spread to lymph nodes, and their treatment and prognosis are usually quite different. Even when lymphoma is diagnosed, it is critical that you and your doctors know just what type of lymphoma you are dealing with. Aggressive lymphomas can take your life quickly but are often cured by chemotherapy, while other types of lymphoma are not curable, but usually take years before they become a problem requiring therapy.

An accurate diagnosis helps you and your family understand what to expect and how to prepare for the future, even if you cannot get curative treatment. Knowing the diagnosis also helps your doctor treat your symptoms better. Many people find "not knowing" very hard, and are relieved when they finally have an explanation for their symptoms. Sometimes a frail patient is obviously dying, and diagnostic studies can be an additional burden; in such cases, it may be quite reasonable to focus on symptom relief (palliation) without knowing the details of the diagnosis.

2. KNOW YOUR CANCER'S STAGE

The cancer's stage defines your prognosis and treatment options. No one can make informed decisions without it. However, just as there may be times when the burdens of diagnostic studies may be too great, it may also be appropriate to do without full staging in very frail, dying patient.

As it is in younger patients, stage is usually determined by the size of the tumor, the presence or absence of cancer in local or regional lymph nodes, and its metastasis to other organs. Most solid tumors are staged using the TNM criteria. When doctors combine this information with information regarding your cancer's specific histology, grade, and other characteristics (for example, tumor receptor status in breast cancer), they can predict what impact, if any, your cancer is likely to have on your life expectancy and quality of life.

3. KNOW YOUR LIFE EXPECTANCY

Anticancer treatment should be considered if you are likely to live long enough to experience symptoms or premature death from your cancer. If your life expectancy is so short that the cancer will not significantly affect it, there may be no reason to aggressively treat your cancer. Palliative treatment may or may not be warranted.

Chronological age (how old you are) should not be the only thing that decides how your cancer should, or should not, be treated. Despite advanced age, people who are relatively healthy often have a life expectancy that is longer than their life expectancy with their cancer. The average 70-year-old woman is likely to live another 16 years, and the average 70-year-old man another 12 years. An 85-year-old person can expect to live an additional 5 to 6 years, and remain independent for most of that time. Even an unhealthy 75-year-old man or woman probably will live 5 to 6 more years; long enough to suffer symptoms and early death from active or recurrent cancer.

4. UNDERSTAND THE GOALS

THE GOALS OF TREATMENT

It is important to be clear whether the goal of treatment is cure (for early or locally-advanced cancer) or palliation (for incurable, advanced, metastatic cancer). If the goal is palliation, you need to understand whether the treatment plan will extend your life, control your symptoms, or both. How likely is it to achieve these goals, and how long will you enjoy the benefits?

When the goal of treatment is palliation, chemotherapy should never be administered without defined endpoints and timelines. It should be clear to everyone what is considered success, how success will be determined (for example, with a symptom controlled or a smaller mass on CAT scan), and by when the success must be achieved. You and your family should understand what your options are at each step and how likely each is to meet your goals. If this is not clear, ask your oncology provider to explain it in words that you understand.

THE GOALS OF THE PATIENT

In addition to the traditional goals of tumor response, increased survival, and symptom control, older cancer patients often have goals related to quality of life. These may include physical and intellectual independence, spending quality time with your family, taking trips, staying out of the hospital, or even economic stability. At times, palliative care or hospice may meet these goals better than active anticancer treatment. In addition to the medical team, older patients often turn to family, friends, and clergy to help guide them.

5. DETERMINE IF YOU ARE FIT OR FRAIL

Deciding how to treat cancer in an older patient requires a thorough understanding of his or her general health and social situation. Decisions about cancer treatment should never focus on age alone.

AGE IS NOT A NUMBER

Your actual age (chronological age) has limited influence on how the cancer will respond to therapy or its prognosis.

Biological and other changes associated with aging are more reliable in estimating an individual's vigor, life expectancy, or the likelihood of treatment complications. These changes include malnutrition; depression; dementia; falls; social isolation; and loss of muscle mass and strength, and the ability to accomplish daily activities such as dressing, bathing, eating, shopping, housekeeping, and managing one's finances or medication.

CHRONIC ILLNESSES

Older cancer patients are likely to have comorbidities that affect their life expectancy; the more illnesses that you have and the more severe the symptoms associated with these illnesses, the greater their effect on your ability to tolerate cancer therapies. This effect has very little impact on the behavior of the cancer itself, but studies do show that comorbidity has a major impact on treatment outcome and its side effects.

6. BALANCE BENEFITS AND HARMS

Fit older cancer patients respond to treatment similarly to their younger counterparts. However, a word of caution: Until recently, few studies included older individuals, and it may not be appropriate to apply these findings to the diverse group of older cancer patients.

The side effects of cancer treatment are never less in the elderly. In addition to the standard side effects, there are significant age-related toxicities to consider. Though most of these are more a function of frailty than chronological age, even the fittest senior cannot avoid the physical effects of aging. In addition to the changes in fat and muscle that you see in the mirror, there are age-related changes in your kidney, liver, and digestive (gastrointestinal) function; these changes affect how your body absorbs and metabolizes anticancer drugs and other medicines. The average older man or woman takes many different medicines (to control, for example, high blood pressure, high cholesterol, osteoporosis, diabetes, and arthritis), and the combination of these multiple medications, or "polypharmacy," can cause undesirable side effects when these drugs interact with each other and the anticancer medications.

7. GET INVOLVED

Healthcare providers and family members often underestimate the physical and mental abilities of older people and their willingness to face chronic and life-threatening conditions. Studies clearly show that older patients want detailed and easily understood information about potential treatments and alternatives. Patients and families may consider cancer untreatable in the aged and not understand the possibilities offered by treatment.

While patients with dementia pose a unique challenge, they are frequently capable of participating in goal setting and simple discussions about treatment side effects and logistics. Caring family members and friends are often able to share the patient's life story so that healthcare workers can work with them to make decisions consistent with the patient's values and desires. This, of course, is no substitute for a well thought-out and properly executed living will or healthcare proxy.

While it is hard to face the possibility of life-threatening events at any age, it is always better to be prepared and to put your affairs in order. In addition to estate planning and wills, it is critical that you outline your wishes regarding medical care at the end of life, and make legal provisions for someone to make those decisions if you are unable to make them for yourself.

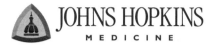

CHAPTER 4

CANCER TREATMENT
IN THE ELDERLY

BY MYA S. THEIN, MD; ILENE S. BROWNER,
MD; AND GARY R. SHAPIRO, MD

---

reatment for your cancer may include some or all of the following approaches: surgery, chemotherapy, radiation therapy, hormonal therapy, targeted therapy, immunotherapy, and other therapies such as a bone marrow transplant or interventional radiology procedures. Cancer treatment can be either curative or palliative. Even if your cancer cannot be cured, treatment can improve your quality and length of life.

Your current medical conditions, functional status, medications, and most importantly, your goals and wishes will impact your treatment plan. This plan will be based on your specific type of cancer, its stage, and its cellular and biologic characteristics, which are discussed in detail in the cancer-specific books of the *Johns Hopkins Patients' Guide* series.

Chapter 3 of this book outlines Seven Practical Steps to help you make decisions about your treatment. It emphasizes that the management of cancer in the older person should not be based on chronological age, but rather on an individualized assessment of each person's physiological age and overall health. This is determined, in part, by a Comprehensive Geriatric Assessment (CGA).

A CGA is an in-depth, multidimensional evaluation that includes an assessment of performance status (functional capacity), life expectancy, concurrent health problems, organ function, nutritional status, memory, mood, medication usage, and socioeconomic and emotional issues. The CGA provides an estimate of your physiological age and overall fitness as it relates to your cancer and its impact on these characteristics. It helps your healthcare provider to determine an individualized, coordinated treatment plan for you. This plan is intended to give you the most therapeutic benefit while minimizing risks and side effects.

This chapter is designed to provide you with an overview of treatment options for cancer. Please refer to the cancer-specific books in the *Johns Hopkins Patients' Guide Series* for details about the treatment of *your* cancer.

SURGERY

When you are diagnosed with cancer, your first encounter with a medical professional is often with a surgeon. Surgeons can be generalists, or they can specialize in surgical oncology or a specific organ system (e.g., a urologist for genitourinary tract disease). A surgeon may be consulted to perform a diagnostic (e.g., excisional biopsy or exploratory surgery to stage your disease), palliative (e.g., a diverting colostomy to bypass a bowel obstruction or a laminectomy to relieve a spinal cord compression), supportive (e.g., indwelling venous catheters or feeding tubes), or curative (e.g., mastectomy) procedure for your cancer.

In most cases, regardless of a patient's age, surgery offers definitive local control of your disease and the best chance for cure if your cancer is removed at an early stage before it has spread to other organs. Examples of curative surgery include nephrectomy for renal cell carcinoma and colectomy for colon cancer. Curative surgery may be performed before or after other treatment(s) for your cancer. Curative surgery is not an option for blood cancers including leukemia, lymphoma, and multiple myeloma or, with few exceptions, for metastatic disease.

The type of surgical procedure performed and the extent of surgery are based on your tumor type, its location, and its clinical stage. Surgery may be the only treatment you need for your cancer (such as in early stage melanoma), or it may be coupled with chemotherapy and/or radiation therapy (e.g., breast cancer). Some patients will not have surgery as part of their cancer care.

Although surgery may be complex, it is as effective in elderly patients as in younger patients, but it does have a somewhat higher rate of complications in older individuals who have other medical problems, or comorbidities. Like other treatment options, surgery in some older individuals may involve risks related to decreases in body organ function, especially the heart and lungs. It is essential that the surgeon and anesthetist work closely with your primary care physician or a consultant to fully assess and treat these problems before, during, and after the operation. In some cases, less-invasive procedures, such as minimally invasive (laparoscopic) surgery or radiofrequency ablation of a mass may be an option for frail individuals or those with a very high surgical risk.

The decision to operate should not be made on the basis of your chronological age, but rather on your physiological age (how fit you are). Because of changes in baseline organ function and an increased number and severity of other medical problems, older patients may have an increased risk for adverse events in the operative period as compared to younger cancer patients. The surgical team will work with your primary care provider and other consultants to optimize your health and minimize your risks. Many hospitals have a geriatric consultation service available for the pre- and postoperative assessment of older patients. Your preoperative evaluation will likely include a more extensive review of your current health problems and symptoms, functional status, social support network, and cognitive status. If time permits, you may be asked to participate in a physical, cognitive, pulmonary, or cardiac rehabilitation program in order to improve your fitness prior to your surgery. With proper assessment, as well as prevention and correction of risk factors for adverse outcomes (e.g., low blood count, low albumin, or dehydration), the older cancer patient can achieve a good surgical outcome.

RADIATION THERAPY

Most cancer patients will receive some radiation therapy during the course of their disease. Radiation therapy is a well-tolerated treatment that uses energy (ionizing radiation) to destroy cancer cells or to reduce the size of your cancer. The goal of radiation therapy is to obtain local control of your cancer, while limiting the damage to nearby normal tissues. It can have a curative, preventive, or palliative role in your prescribed treatment plan. It can be given alone or combined with surgery, chemotherapy, or hormonal or targeted therapy. Radiation can be given before the surgery to shrink the size of your cancer (neoadjuvant therapy), or after the surgery to prevent recurrence (adjuvant therapy) or to kill any remaining cancer cells. In advanced cancer, radiation therapy can relieve your symptoms and improve your quality of life.

If radiation therapy is recommended as part of your treatment plan, you will be referred to a radiation oncologist. Before you begin your treatment, you will have a pretreatment CAT scan performed to locate the tumor and identify the surrounding normal tissue. The CAT scan also will be used to simulate your treatment position and generate a treatment map and dose. Non-permanent marks will be placed on your skin to insure proper positioning when you return for your actual treatment. Your radiation may be delivered by any of the following methods:

- *External beam radiation.* External beam radiation is delivered from a machine outside of your body. Total dose and duration depends on the type and size of your cancer, as well as your general health and other concurrent treatments. It is usually a painless procedure and lasts 15–30 minutes.

- *Internal radiation.* Internal radiation, or brachytherapy, is delivered by radioactive seeds or pellets placed inside of your body and within or close to your tumor. It may be used for localized prostate cancer, cervical or uterine cancer, lung cancer, and head and neck cancers. The procedure is usually performed in a hospital operating room under anesthesia.

- *Intraoperative radiation.* Intraoperative radiation involves external beam radiation being given directly to the tumor or tumor bed during surgery.

- *Stereotactic surgery.* Stereotactic surgery is a 3-dimensional technique that delivers a large dose of radiation to a tumor field in one or more fractions. It is used in the treatment of brain tumors, and increasingly, for patients at high-risk for surgical intervention or for tumors deemed inoperable. Cyberknife or gammaknife radiosurgery are types of stereotactic radiotherapy.

- *Systemic radiation therapy.* Systemic radiation therapy involves injecting radioactive substances into a vein to deliver radiation to multiple sites or a large area of disease. It is often used for the treatment of thyroid cancer or painful, diffusely metastatic bone lesions.

Radiation therapy is well-tolerated by older adults and can often control disease or symptoms in patients who are not able to tolerate a surgical intervention or systemic therapy due to their other health conditions. However, the frequency of treatment visits and treatment-related side effects may be more problematic for the older patient. Since radiation therapy is typically given daily over a period of weeks, transportation to and from the radiation center may be difficult for an older patient who no longer drives, has limited functional mobility, or little social support. If transportation is an issue, talk with a social worker at your radiation center; he or she may be able to identify resources to assist you. If severe arthritis, weakness from a stroke, or other disabilities make it difficult for you to get around, talk to your primary care provider or radiation oncologist about physical and occupational therapy or assistive devices. Improving your mobility will make getting back and forth to your daily appointments a bit easier for you and your caregivers.

Radiation therapy can cause treatment-related side effects such as skin burns, swallowing problems and pain due to esophagitis (inflammation and irritation of the esophagus), diarrhea, and less commonly, low blood counts or loss of bone density. Although temporary and treatable, these symptoms are usually more problematic in older patients who have concurrent health problems and age-related changes in their organ function. Symptoms may be prevented or minimized with careful monitoring.

Fatigue is also a common side effect of radiation therapy and may be more pronounced in older patients. Fatigue arises from a combination of the treatment itself, its associated side effects, and the daily visits. It is important to get plenty of rest during your treatment. Participation in light exercise may help to limit your fatigue. If you experience crushing fatigue, talk to your provider.

Older patients receiving radiation to their brain are more susceptible to radiation-induced memory problems and cognitive decline than younger patients. These changes can occur immediately, or over the following months or years. An assessment of your cognitive function should be performed prior to receiving radiation therapy to the brain in order to identify any deficits in your memory or thinking, as well as after therapy to identify any treatment-related changes. Your memory or mood may also be affected by the corticosteroids that are often given to patients receiving radiation therapy to their brain and spine. Good control of your blood pressure and blood sugar, light exercise, and performance of cognitive tasks such as puzzles may minimize the impact of radiation therapy on your brain.

INTERVENTIONAL RADIOLOGY PROCEDURES

Specially-trained radiologists may perform minimally invasive procedures using image guidance (CAT scans or ultrasound) to treat your cancer or to improve your quality of life by decreasing symptoms. Older patients who are at high risk for operative procedures may be good candidates for interventional approaches. The following interventional procedures are available:

- *Chemoembolization.* Chemoembolization delivers chemotherapy drugs directly into the tumor via the bloodstream (such as for treatment of metastatic liver lesions or liver cancer).

- *Tumor ablation.* Tumor ablation kills cancer cells by the application of heat, freezing cold, microwaves, or other substances via a special catheter inserted directly into the tumor.

- *Stents and drains.* A stent or drain can be placed under image guidance to relieve an obstruction in your bowel, liver, or bladder. Placement often relieves pain and prevents complications such as infection.

- *Indwelling venous catheters.* A catheter may be placed to deliver medications, fluids, or blood products. Other catheters also may be used to drain symptomatic fluid accumulations from your lung (pleural effusion), abdomen (ascites), or bladder.

- *Kyphoplasty.* Kyphoplasty is a procedure performed to stabilize a compression fracture in a bone in your spine, which may also help to relieve pain and maintain physical function.

- *Filters.* A filter may be placed in a vein if you have a blood clot and are unable to take blood thinners.

- *Nerve blocks.* Nerve blocks relieve localized pain via an injection of numbing medicine into a nerve. It is often used to treat pain from pancreatic or cervical cancer.

SYSTEMIC THERAPY

In contrast to radiation therapy and surgery, which affect only a specific area of the body, systemic treatments travel through the blood stream to affect the whole body. They are used to alter the activity, growth, and survival of your cancer cells wherever they may be in your body. They are most often given intravenously, but some systemic agents are designed to enter the blood stream after they are taken by mouth or injected with a needle into the muscle or the skin. Although the term "chemotherapy" is commonly used as a catch-all term for systemic therapies, the term properly refers to cytotoxic therapy, a very specific type of systemic treatment. Other types of systemic treatment include: hormonal therapy, immunotherapy, and targeted therapy. Non-frail older cancer patients respond to systemic therapy similarly to their younger counterparts.

Systemic therapy is often an essential part of the treatment of most solid and hematological cancers. It can be given as a single agent or in combination regimens. It is an important adjunct to surgery in patients whose tumors have been completely removed, but who are at risk for recurrence. It also may be a useful and effective option for controlling symptoms and increasing longevity in non-frail seniors with advanced or metastatic cancer.

Both palliative and curative systemic therapy can be used alone or concurrent with or sequential to surgery or radiation. If your systemic therapy is given before your surgery, it is called neoadjuvant therapy. The goal of neoadjuvant therapy is to shrink your cancer in order to decrease surgical risk and operative time, improve likelihood of a complete resection, and minimize deformity. If your systemic therapy is administered after your surgery, it is called adjuvant therapy. The primary aim of adjuvant therapy is to destroy any circulating, undetectable (microscopic) cancer cells and to prevent a future recurrence of your cancer. Systemic therapy also can be administered concurrent with radiation in either sensitizing doses to improve the penetration of the radiation (as for rectal cancer) or treatment doses (as for inoperable but curable non-small cell lung cancer).

TYPES OF SYSTEMIC THERAPY

Cytotoxic therapy. Chemotherapy agents are classified by their mechanism of action. Some agents kill cancer cells by impairing their function or interfering with DNA activity. Other agents work by altering cancer cell division or by competing with nutrients that the cancer cells need for growth and survival.

Your cancer may be treated with a single drug or a combination of drugs; the efficacy of your treatment regimen is not always directly associated with the number of chemotherapy agents you receive. Multi-agent regimens combine drugs with different mechanisms of action and nonoverlapping side effects in order to maximize the treatment of your cancer while minimizing side effects.

Although older patients may have more chronic medical problems and may have underlying age-associated changes in their organ function, clinical trials have shown that non-frail older cancer patients often tolerate chemotherapy as well as younger patients. Careful monitoring for symptoms and early intervention are critical to limiting side effects and insuring successful receipt of chemotherapy. Reducing the dose of chemotherapy based purely on chronological age may seriously affect the effectiveness of treatment. On the other hand, older patients may need lower doses if they have reduced kidney or liver function. Managing chemotherapy-associated toxicity with appropriate supportive care is crucial in the elderly population to ensure the best chance of cure and survival or to provide the best palliation.

Older cancer patients have higher rates of fatigue, mucositis (mouth sores), diarrhea, neutropenia, thrombocytopenia, and anemia, as well as heart (cardiotoxicity), liver (hepatotoxicity), and kidney (nephrotoxicity) side effects.

Though the side effects of cancer treatment are potentially more burdensome in the elderly, they can be managed by oncologists, especially geriatric oncologists, who work in teams with others who specialize in the care of the elderly. With appropriate care, healthy older patients do just as well with chemotherapy as younger patients. Advances in supportive care (antinausea medicines and blood cell growth factors) have significantly decreased the side effects of chemotherapy, and improved safety and the quality of life of individuals with cancer. Nonetheless, there is risk, especially if the patient is frail. The presence of severe comorbidities, age-related frailty, or underlying severe psychosocial problems may be obstacles for highly-intensive treatment plans. Such patients may benefit from less complicated or potentially less toxic treatment plans.

When choosing a palliative chemotherapy regimen, preference should be given to chemotherapeutic drugs with safer profiles. Single agent therapy is less toxic than, and probably just as effective as, combination chemotherapy in the treatment of most metastatic cancers.

Hormonal therapy. Hormonal therapy is used to treat cancers of the breast, prostate, and uterus. Hormones can stimulate the growth of these tumors, and the goal of hormonal therapy is to block this growth pathway. Blockade can be done surgically by removing a hormone-producing or responding organ, such as the ovary or testis, or pharmacologically by administering medications that block hormonal receptors in the responding organ (breast or prostate) or stop organs such as the adrenal glands from producing their stimulatory hormones. Hormonal medications include selective estrogen receptor modulators, aromatase inhibitors (AI), antiandrogens, and agents that disrupt the activity of luteinizing hormone.

Hormonal therapy is a relatively safe therapy. Common side effects may include hot flashes, fatigue, mood changes, weight gain, loss of desire for sexual relations, and sexual dysfunction. Women may experience vaginal dryness and irritation, and men may experience enlargement of their breasts. Some hormonal therapy may affect your cholesterol level, and you should have a baseline fasting cholesterol panel checked at the initiation of and during your therapy, especially if you have a history of diabetes, hypertension, or heart disease. Vascular events such as strokes or blood clots are a rare side effect of hormonal therapy.

Since older patients are likely to be less mobile and to partake in less exercise, get less sun exposure, have less calcium-rich diets, and have other health problems such as hypothyroidism and take medications (diuretics) that affect their bone density, they are at greater risk for bone loss (osteopenia or osteoporosis) with certain hormonal therapies. If you are prescribed hormonal therapy for your cancer, you should have a baseline bone density (DEXA) scan performed. You also should have your vitamin D level checked and, if low, repleted. Patients on hormonal therapy should take calcium and vitamin D supplements as recommended by their provider. If your bone density is low, your provider may prescribe an oral or intravenous bisphosphonate to strengthen your bones and help prevent a fracture of your hip or spine.

Immunotherapy. Immunotherapy, also known as biologic therapy, stimulates the immune system to prevent or treat cancer. Currently available drugs include recombinant interferon-α (rIFN-α) for the treatment of blood cancers, kidney cancer and melanoma, and interleukin-2 (IL-2) for the treatment of kidney cancer and melanoma. High doses of IL-2 are not typically prescribed for older patients because of its significant side effect profile. rIFN-α has been studied in older patients with cancer, and at low doses, it appears to be well-tolerated in all patients regardless of age. Side effects may include mood changes, low grade fevers, and flu-like symptoms. Thalomid (thalidomide) and Revlimid (lenalidomide) are immunomodulatory agents used primarily in the treatment of multiple myeloma. Side effects of Thalomid include fatigue, constipation, neuropathy, and an increased risk for blood clots. Older patients with diabetes or vascular disease may be more likely to experience these side effects. Revlimid is better tolerated but can be associated with pronounced myelosuppression, especially in older patients.

Targeted therapy. Targeted therapy is a type of treatment that targets a specific tumor pathway or a protein or gene required for tumor growth. Targeted therapies include biological response modifiers and agents that disrupt the cell-signaling pathways that affect tumor growth and survival.

The biological response modifiers include the monoclonal antibodies Rituxan (rituximab), Avastin (bevacizumab) and Herceptin (trastuzumab). These agents can be associated with significant infusion-related reactions and cardiac toxicity, including hypersensitivity/allergic reactions, arrhythmias, acute myocardial infarction or heart failure, and elevated blood pressure. Rituxan is used primarily for the treatment non-Hodgkin's lymphoma, and can be used as a single agent or combined with chemotherapy. Herceptin targets the HER2neu receptors overexpressed in some types of breast cancer, and is typically used in combination with chemotherapy. Avastin inhibits blood vessel formation within a tumor, and is used with chemotherapy in the treatment of advanced breast, colon, and non-small cell lung cancers.

Inhibitors of cell signaling pathways or receptors include tyrosine kinase inhibitors (TKI) such as Erbitux (cetuximab), Gleevec (imatinib), Tarceva (erlotinib), Sutent (sunitinib), or Nexavar (sorafenib), and the motor inhibitors such as Afinitor (everolimus). TKIs are administered orally and daily, except for Erbitux, which is administered intravenously and weekly. These agents are used in the treatment of both solid and hematologic malignancies. TKI side effects include a skin rash on the face and chest, diarrhea, mouth sores, cough, hypertension, interactions with Coumadin (warfarin; a blood thinner), and a slight increased risk of thromboarterial events. Direct damage to the heart is possible, but uncommon. Side effects of the motor inhibitors include hypertension, a decrease in heart function, mouth sores, and a fall in blood counts.

Because of their antitumor-specific action, targeted therapies may have fewer side effects than other forms of treatment. Older patients, however, may be more susceptible to some of these adverse effects, including the heart toxicity associated with Herceptin, the diarrhea and electrolyte changes associated with Erbitux, and the bleeding and vascular events associated with Avastin.

OTHER CANCER TREATMENTS

Bone marrow transplant or stem cell transplant. Bone marrow or stem cell transplantation is sometimes used to treat certain types of leukemia (chronic myelogenous leukemia [CML], myelodysplastic syndrome [MDS], and acute leukemia especially when acute myelogenous leukemia [AML] or acute lymphocytic leukemia [ALL] is refractory to standard treatment) and multiple myeloma. It is also used to treat some lymphomas or those that are refractory to standard treatment. Stem cell transplantation is a complex procedure that requires a multidisciplinary team of physicians, nurses, social workers, and ancillary staff. It requires meticulous planning, and is typically done in tertiary centers. There are 2 types of stem cell transplant. An autologous stem cell transplant uses cells provided from the patient, whereas allogeneic transplants use cells from a family member or a tissue typed unrelated donor. In both autologous and allogeneic transplants, very high doses of chemotherapy are used to kill the malignant cells. The dose of chemotherapy is so high that it also kills the normal bone marrow (or stem cells). The stem cells that are harvested from the patient (autologous) or donor (allogeneic) are used to rescue the patient's normal bone marrow by replanting it with stem cells so that it will function normally. Allogeneic transplant also produces an immunologic effect that works to kill the leukemia or lymphoma cells. Given the complexities, and importance of careful monitoring, most patients require hospitalization for about a month for the procedure, and close follow up afterwards.

These are extremely risky procedures, even in the young and healthy. The risks increase dramatically with greater age and are usually over the top if you have any significant comorbidity. It used to be said that anyone over 50 years old should not have a transplant, but recent advances now make it possible for carefully selected fit seniors to consider these forms of aggressive therapy, especially the autologous type of transplant procedure. Although the risks of standard allogeneic transplant are usually too great for any older person, some transplant centers include the fit elderly in their "mini transplant" (nonmyeloablative stem cell transplants) research studies.

Clinical trials. Clinical trials are research studies in which new drugs or procedures are evaluated to determine if a treatment is safe and effective, and if it offers similar or better outcomes then current regimens. Clinical trials are designed with patient safety in mind! Although the incidence of cancer in the elderly is high, older patients are woefully underrepresented in clinical trials for new cancer treatments. Historically, older patients were not enrolled in clinical trials for a number of reasons, including chronological age and strict exclusion criteria such as poor functional status, chronic health problems, and memory impairment. The National Institute of Aging and the NCI now support clinical trials specifically designed to address the treatment needs of the older adult and have encouraged less stringent exclusion criteria. During the course of your therapy, you may be offered the opportunity to participate in a clinical trial.

Most clinical trials are conducted in phases. There are three phases of clinical trials designed to assess the safety, toxicity, efficacy, and effectiveness of the drugs or procedures under investigation. Each phase builds on the information obtained from the previous phase. Your eligibility for a given trial phase is dependent on your cancer stage and available treatments, as well as treatments already received.

CONCLUSION

The challenge of cancer care in the older patient is to determine the balance between the benefits and risks of treatment. There are three questions that need to be answered before starting any treatment: (1) Will your longevity be compromised by your cancer?; (2) Will you tolerate the side effects of treatment?; and (3) How will your cancer and its treatment affect your daily function, quality of life, and longevity?

The first question addresses your type of cancer and its stage, as well as the effectiveness of available treatments. It also addresses whether or not you have concurrent health problems that might limit your life expectancy independent of your cancer, or make your cancer treatment less tolerable or less effective. Whether or not you will tolerate your cancer treatment(s) depends, in part, on your other health problems, and your cognitive and physical functioning. A thorough evaluation of your global health, quality of life, and socioeconomic status can detect issues that may render you more susceptible to treatment toxicity and determine your fitness for therapy. Addressing and correcting these issues, prior to and throughout your cancer treatment, can render you more fit for therapy, and limit the risks and increase the benefit of your treatments. In addition to the answers to these questions, your personal preferences and goals should be taken into consideration when determining your fitness for therapy and when generating a disease and stage specific, individualized treatment plan that meets all of your needs.

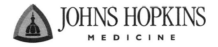

CHAPTER 5

Biology of Aging and Cancer Treatment

By Madelaine Binner, DNP, MBA, CRNP-BC

Geriatric oncology is a sub-specialty of oncology that deals with the comprehensive health care of older persons with a diagnosis of cancer. As a person moves from middle age through later life, the body undergoes many changes. These changes impact the physiological, sociological, psychological, and functional aspects of a person's response to cancer and its treatment(s).

Compared to younger individuals, those over 65 years of age are at a higher risk for cancer. Cancer is a disease of aging, and its incidence is increasing as people live longer. Several explanations for the association between cancer and aging have been suggested; some of which include: the older person has had a more prolonged exposure to carcinogens; the internal cellular environment of the aged adult is more favorable for cancer cell growth; and a combination of carcinogenic exposure and favorable internal conditions that enhance genetic tendency for abnormal cell growth.

Physiologic changes associated with aging, such as a less-efficient immune system, are particularly pertinent to cancer and its treatment. Chronological age may be associated with the physiological changes of aging, but age alone should not determine cancer treatment options for an older patient. Considerations in decision making need to include the overall health of the patient, the patient's ability to tolerate the stress of anti-cancer therapy, and if treatment will provide more benefit than harm. It is essential to address the specific needs of each older person with cancer in order to achieve the best clinical response while maintaining a good quality of life.

In this chapter, the major physiological changes associated with the aging process and how these changes may impact the geriatric oncology patient's treatment and response to treatment are discussed.

BLOOD AND IMMUNE SYSTEMS

The blood and immune systems are closely related and basically consist of red blood cells, white blood cells, platelets, bone marrow, the spleen, and lymph nodes. The risk and severity of chemotherapy effects on these blood and immune system components increase with age. Myelosuppression is a condition in which bone marrow activity is decreased, resulting in fewer red blood cells, white blood cells, and platelets. It is a common side effect of some cancers and some cancer treatments. Strain on the blood cell production system may overwhelm the older patient's limited cell reserve, and thus the ability to compensate for this additional burden. Symptoms of fatigue, increased heart rate, and shortness of breath may develop if red blood cell production is reduced, a condition known as anemia. Alternatively, if white blood cell counts drop or platelets are reduced, the geriatric oncology patient may be at increased risk for infection or bleeding, respectively.

With advancing age, a person is more susceptible to infection, illness, and disease and there is often a longer recovery period after an acute incident. The immune system, which is the body's protection against illness and infection, is not as efficient and is less sensitive to reacting to signals in the body that indicate a problem. Infection-fighting cells (white blood cells) tend to be weaker and the duration of their protective ability is shortened. Cancer treatments, such as radiation and chemotherapy, further stress the already vulnerable immune system in the aged. Fortunately, there are medications currently available to treat myelosuppression caused by cancer treatment. These drugs can stimulate the production of red or white blood cells to assist the older patient through periods when blood counts may be exceptionally low.

HEART AND BLOOD VESSELS

The amount of blood pumped by the heart per minute (cardiac output) decreases as a person ages. The normal adult heart pumps about five quarts of blood per minute when at rest. In a person without any heart disease, there is approximately a 1% per year decrease in cardiac output after age 30. Blood pressure increases, with the most notable increase in the systolic blood pressure. Arteries become more rigid and veins are less efficient in returning blood flow to the heart. Atherosclerosis (or clogging of the arteries with fatty deposits and cholesterol) has been shown to clearly increase with age. In addition to changes in the heart's muscle action (pump) and blood flow (vessels), there may be alterations in the heart's electrical system, resulting in an increased risk of irregular heartbeats (arrhythmias).

Anthracyclines, a group of chemotherapy agents that includes Adriamycin (doxorubicin), and chest radiation treatments have the potential to weaken heart muscle cells. The medical term for this condition is called cardiomyopathy. Radiation treatments to the chest may also impact the functioning of heart valves and coronary arteries.

Herceptin, a drug often used for treating breast cancer that has an excessive growth protein known as HER2neu, has been associated with weakening of the heart muscle when given over time. Another targeted therapy, Avastin, is used in the treatment of advanced cancers such as metastatic colorectal, renal, breast, and lung cancers. It may increase the risks for hypertension, blood clot formation, hemorrhage, and stroke. Because of the physiologic changes associated with the aging process and preexisting medical conditions (like diabetes, chronic obstructive lung disease, heart disease, and congestive heart failure), the risk of developing these complications may be more pronounced in the older person, and the ability to compensate for these cardiac changes may be diminished. These side effects may be minimized with close monitoring of heart function during treatment. Your oncologist may order an electrocardiogram (ECG, sometimes called EKG) to rule out underlying irregular heart rhythms or prior injury to your heart, as well as a MUGA (multiple-gated acquisition nuclear scan of heart function) scan or an echocardiogram (ECHO or ultrasound of the heart) to check the heart's ability to pump blood effectively. Your surgical oncologist also may refer you to a heart specialist before surgery, so that your heart health can be evaluated to prevent any unexpected heart complications during or following your surgery.

LUNGS

The amount of air the lungs can inhale and exhale decreases with age. The lungs become more rigid and the exchange of oxygen is also less efficient. The older person has a less-effective cough reflex and the ability to handle physical challenges, such as running or stair climbing, is reduced. As part of the aging process, the chest wall becomes less flexible and the immune system becomes less effective. These changes render older individuals more prone to pneumonia and other lung infections. Indeed, this reduced lung function is further compromised if a patient has a history of asthma or chronic obstructive lung disease.

A less-effective respiratory system impacts the postoperative recovery of the aging adult. If the older patient can be physiologically and psychologically prepared for anticipated surgery, postoperative mortality and complications may be minimized. Your doctor may ask you to have PFTs (pulmonary function tests) or a Ventilation-Perfusion (V/Q) scan to evaluate your lung function and gas exchange prior to surgery, especially lung or chest surgery. It is imperative that the older patient performs coughing and deep-breathing exercises following surgery, refrains from smoking before and after the surgical operation, and begins physical activity as soon as possible after any invasive procedure. Surgical treatment for cancer in the older adult is associated with increased mortality and postoperative complications; however, risks associated with *elective surgery* are minimally increased in the aged. This factor supports the notion that cancer screening in the aged should continue to be considered in their healthcare management. Also, advances in anesthesia and alternative procedures, such as tumor ablation (see Chapter 4), may offer the older patient safe and effective management of their disease.

KIDNEYS AND BLADDER

A gradual decrease in the volume and weight of the kidneys occurs with aging. Kidney size in a 90-year-old person is about 70% of that of a 30-year-old. There is also a decline in the number of functioning units in the kidney, which rids the body of wastes, water, and drugs (medications). In persons younger than 65-years-old, the bladder can hold about 2 cups of urine, compared to about 1 cup for those age 65 and older. The bladder becomes smaller and less expandable, resulting in frequent urination and nocturia (awakening during the night to urinate, thus interrupting sleep); has a reduced ability to contract, causing hesitancy with urination; and has reduced control over suppression of bladder contractions, leading to a sense of urgency. There may also be a delay in the sensation of the need to urinate, often resulting in urinary incontinence. In older men, the prostate gland often enlarges and impedes the free flow of urine. Many older people may be on medications such as diuretics, blood pressure medications, and treatments for overactive bladder, which may further complicate kidney and urinary function. A major consideration in the treatment of cancer in an older person is kidney function, because many chemotherapy drugs and other medications used in the treatment of cancer are excreted by the kidneys. Also, some chemotherapy agents, such as Platinol-AQ (cisplatin), may be potentially harmful to the kidneys. Some chemotherapy doses are calculated based on kidney function and must be adjusted to address the reduced renal function associated with aging.

GASTROINTESTINAL SYSTEM

Decreases in saliva, resulting in dry mouth, dental decay, inflammation of the gums (gingivitis), and a decreased sense of taste and smell, may contribute to inadequate nutrition. Swallowing may be impaired due to disturbances in the ability of the esophagus to move food down to the stomach, as well as a prior stroke. The stomach may be slower in the digestive process because of a decrease in production of gastric juices needed to digest foods, or the use of antacid medications. The small intestine may be limited in its ability to absorb certain nutrients such as calcium, vitamin B12, and folic acid. Intestinal motility is reduced with age and other conditions, such as with diabetes. The colon has less tone, leading to increased storage and dehydration of the stool in the bowel, which results in constipation. There is a reduction in the weight of the liver by as much as 20% after the age of 50; in an elderly person, certain drugs are known to be metabolized (processed) more slowly by the liver, and this may change their effectiveness and side-effect profile.

Gastrointestinal side effects of many chemotherapy agents and radiation therapy increase the older person's need for nutritional support during cancer treatment, and taste changes and diminished appetite may develop in some patients. To maintain an adequate nutritional status, a multivitamin or high-calorie protein supplements, such as Boost or Ensure, may be recommended. Oral mucositis (inflammation of the mucous membranes of the mouth), a common side effect of some treatments, is managed with prescribed oral rinses, good dental hygiene, and the use of a soft toothbrush. Pre- and post-therapy antinausea medications are often used to manage nausea and vomiting side effects. Many anti-cancer drugs, such as Xeloda (capecitabine) may induce diarrhea, which can result in dehydration. Diarrhea is often a problem in older patients because of decreased thirst drive, use of diuretics, slowed or limited mobility, and risk for infection. Antidiarrhea medicine, such as Imodium (loperamide), is prescribed to control diarrhea. For patients receiving radiation therapy, especially to the chest, upper airways, or esophagus, nutritional support may be achieved with the insertion of a feeding tube. In the aging person, constipation is not uncommon and the use of narcotic pain medicines may aggravate this condition. Stool softeners and bowel stimulants are recommended to ensure normal bowel patterns in an older patient using narcotics for cancer pain management.

Because of changes in gastrointestinal motility, acid production, and nutrient absorption in an older person, it is unclear if oral chemotherapy agents will be as effectively absorbed and distributed into the systemic circulation. As more oral anti-cancer agents are developed, it is essential to include patients 70 years and older in clinical trials of these agents.

MUSCLES AND BONES

As a person ages, there is a decline in muscle mass and an increase in fat storage in tissue, primarily caused by the loss and shrinkage of muscle cells and an increase in the size of fat cells. Physical activity and exercise is recommended to maintain muscle strength and function and to prevent or reduce obesity. Also, if mobility and physical function are impaired, the risk for developing geriatric syndromes (such as falls, delirium, incontinence, and osteoporosis) increases and the tolerance for cancer treatment decreases. Degenerative joint disease (osteoarthritis) affects 85% of people over the age of 70 and may cause severe disability. This is the "wear and tear" type of joint pain affecting essential weight-bearing joints like your knees. Another skeletal disorder is osteoporosis. This condition leads to weak, fragile bones. Bone mass decreases by 10% per decade for women and 5% per decade for men beginning about the age of 40; this decrease may result in reduction in height, stooped posture, limited mobility, and an increased risk for fractures. Other conditions, such as underactive thyroid treated with Levothroid (levothyroxine) and gastroesophageal reflux disease (indigestion or "heartburn") treated with long-term proton pump inhibitors (medicine that reduce stomach acid), also may lead to bone loss. Older persons may not have adequate intake of calcium and vitamin D in their diets, which is another contributing factor to decreased bone mineral density.

Aromatase inhibitors (AIs) are a class of drugs commonly used for patients with hormone-receptor positive breast cancer. These medications, including Arimidex (anastrozole), Femara (letrozole), and Aromasin (exemestane), are associated with an accelerated bone loss. Post-menopausal women are already at increased risk for developing osteoporosis and subsequent fractures; the addition of a hormonal therapy for cancer, such as an AI, further contributes to bone loss and developing osteoporosis or worsening of the patient's bone health. Other hormonal therapies, including Zoladex (goserelin), Lupron (leuprolide), and Casodex (bicalutamide), are used for treatment of prostate cancer reduce the effects of testosterone and androgens, thereby impacting bone health as well. Bone exposed to radiation treatments are also at increased risk for fractures. Your oncology provider may order a DEXA bone density scan to establish a baseline for monitoring bone health if you are taking an AI for breast cancer, or a hormonal therapy for prostate cancer. In addition, medications to prevent or slow the process of osteoporosis, a class of drugs called bisphosphonates, may be ordered, as well as vitamin D and calcium supplements.

BRAIN AND NERVOUS SYSTEM

There tends to be a slowing in the reaction and response time in the aging person. There is a noticeable decline in the innate ability for learning new knowledge as a person enters middle age; as a result, the older adult may require more time to learn and perform a new task. Acquired intelligence or knowledge gained through experience increases as we age; however, there is a delay in the ability to retrieve stored information. The older learner does better when given more time to organize information, distractions are minimized, and learning is self-paced.

Chemo-brain is a term that has been used to describe the thinking and memory impairments often associated with cancer treatment, though research has not clearly demonstrated that cancer treatments are the direct cause of memory or thought processing decline in older cancer patients. Symptoms such as forgetfulness, disorganization, difficulty concentrating, limited attention span, and short term memory problems, among others, may not necessarily indicate chemo-brain, as some of these same symptoms may be related to the aging process, stress, or other health problems.

Peripheral neuropathy may be another side effect of treatment with some types of chemotherapy agents, such as taxanes, platinum compounds, and vinca alkaloids. Peripheral neuropathy can develop when nerves are exposed to certain chemotherapy drugs. Symptoms may include tingling, burning, prickly sensations in the fingers and toes, sensations of electrical shocks, numbness, loss of sensation, or even abnormal sensation to touch (for instance, exaggerated pain to light touch). These symptoms may be permanent, but tend to diminish with adjusted chemotherapy doses or when treatment is discontinued. Neuropathy may impact the patient's sense of balance, impair the ability to perform simple tasks such as buttoning or zipping clothing, decrease the ability to determine temperature sensation, or delay reaction times to various stimuli. These impairments increase the potential for injury due to falls, frostbite, or burns and may restrict an individual's level of independent functioning with such tasks as dressing, preparing meals, or driving. Older patients who may already have decreased sensation and delayed reflex and reaction times, due to diabetic neuropathy or a history of stroke, for example, may be at an increased risk of injury or functional impairment. It is important that you inform your oncologist or nurse if you develop any of these symptoms before, during, or after the course of any cancer treatment.

SKIN

As the body ages, the skin becomes thinner and drier, loses tone and elasticity, and has a decrease in blood vessels. An older person's skin has a tendency to develop bruises or sores more easily, have diminished sensation, and have more difficulty in maintaining normal temperature. Healing is also impaired; thus, the older person is at higher risk for sustaining skin injuries, infection, and pressure sores. Precautions to prevent complications from some of these skin changes include minimizing skin exposure to sunlight, moisturizing skin, and participating in routine exercise. Use of heating pads and hot water bottles is not advised.

Some chemotherapy drugs are associated with certain skin and nail changes. Some chemotherapy drugs (e.g., Xeloda) may induce a skin condition referred to as hand-foot syndrome. This condition may be characterized by tingling, numbness, pain, redness, dryness, rash, swelling, itching, and darkening of skin of the hands and feet. Intense moisturizing of the skin with products such as lanolin-based or petroleum jelly-based lotions and salves may help in reducing these potential side effects. Other cancer medications, including Erbitux and Tarceva, can cause acne-like, pustular, or blister-like lesions of the skin, along with other skin reactions. Redness, swelling, peeling, dryness, itching, ulcerations, and infection are some of the skin changes commonly seen with cancer radiation treatments.

Extra care should be taken when managing skin care during cancer treatments. Be sure to check with your oncology provider or radiation oncologist for types of products to use and to avoid during treatment. Ice or heat applications should not be used unless prescribed. Sun protection is essential during the course of cancer therapy. Use mild, fragrance-free and alcohol-free soaps and lotions recommended by your oncology professional. Using adhesives on or shaving treated areas should be avoided. Radiation to the genital or rectal areas requires additional precautions; gentle cleansing of this area after bowel movements and the use of sitz baths may decrease the potential for infection and minimize discomfort during and following the treatment period. If your skin changes occur during your treatment, you should bring it to the attention of your cancer professional.

VISION AND HEARING

As we age, visual changes occur in the lenses of the eye. The ability of the eye lens to adjust to near and far vision is significantly decreased. Pupil size decreases with age, requiring more light to accomplish visual tasks. Focusing and color discrimination become less accurate, sensitivity to glare increases, and adapting to changes in light levels is slowed. Eyeglasses and increasing illumination may assist the older person considerably. Glaucoma, cataracts, and macular degeneration are conditions that commonly occur in the older patient. Chemotherapy agents such as Platinol-AQ and steroids, which are often used in cancer therapy, may aggravate these eye problems.

The older person often has difficulty hearing high-pitched sounds. Background noise may interfere with your hearing ability, not only because it is a distraction, but also because the older person must also try and discriminate between these additional sounds. Hearing loss in the aged may result in social isolation and withdrawal, as well as make your treatment more difficult given the potential for lost or misunderstood information. Tell your provider if you are having difficulty hearing them or understanding what they are saying.

Platinol-AQ is an example of a cancer treatment drug that may further impair vision and hearing in the older person. High frequency hearing loss, ringing in the ears, visual disturbances, and altered color perception, although rare, may be observed in some patients. Older adult cancer patients are once again reminded to inform their healthcare providers if any of these symptoms occur.

From this overview, it is apparent that the changes that occur through the aging process are normal, but may be impacted further with the addition of various cancer treatment modalities. As discussed in Chapter 4, it is important for the geriatric cancer patient to have a CGA performed prior to initiation of and periodically throughout one's cancer treatment, in order to distinguish between developing consequences of therapy and the normal aging process.

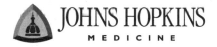

CHAPTER 6

CANCER SURVIVORSHIP

BY ILENE S. BROWNER, MD

WHO IS A SURVIVOR?

Currently, there are more than 10 million cancer survivors in the United States. But who are these survivors? The National Coalition for Cancer Survivorship defines a cancer survivor as an individual with cancer, "from the moment of diagnosis and for the balance of life." However, some patients do not consider themselves to be survivors until after completion of their treatment or after a set period of time without a recurrence, such as a 2- or 5-year anniversary. Family members and friends also may be considered survivors, since they experience the disease and its treatment through the patient.

Many survivors report feeling different after completing their cancer therapy than they did prior to their cancer diagnosis. The cancer experience is transformative. Survivors report both subtle and significant changes in their mood, function, endurance, health, memory and thinking, and social interactions. Some patients feel like they have a new lease on life and are ready to get back to living their lives and tackle the next phase of cancer recovery and surveillance. Other patients have difficulty re-identifying with their non-patient role(s) and activities. They feel uncertain and lost when the flurry of appointments and treatments end. "What next" causes them fear, and they do not trust the transition to wellness. Some express a sense of abandonment, and others have difficulty coping with the uncertainty of treatment benefit and the risk of recurrence. With active treatment, patients often feel safe and protected, but without treatment, they do not have sufficient armor against the ravages of cancer. Strong social support from family and friends, healthcare providers, and community-based programs can reduce stress, enhance quality of life, and provide a buffer for a cancer survivor's active and post-treatment experiences. Older survivors may not have adequate social support or access to support. Engaging in support groups, prior activities or counseling may help to smooth your transition back to health and well-being.

A WELLNESS PLAN FOR SURVIVORS

As you transition from the intervention to the surveillance phase of your cancer care, you will have many questions about your future cancer care. Talk with your oncology provider about the following questions:

- With whom should I get my follow-up care? My oncologist? My primary care provider? My surgeon?

- How often do I need to be seen by my care team?

- What tests and procedures will I need? And how often?

- How quickly will I recover from my treatment?

- What can I do to prevent my cancer from coming back?

- What long-term side effects will I have?

Development of a wellness or survivorship plan at the time of diagnosis can help establish an active pattern of care that will ensure proper coordination of your cancer and general health care, now and in the future, and surveillance for disease recurrence and development of cancer-related side effects or complications.

Coordination between your primary care provider or geriatrician and your other healthcare providers is very important in ensuring continuity of care and well-being. In most cases, you will have a long-term relationship with your oncology provider, who will continue to see you for your post-treatment cancer care. You also may have follow-up appointments scheduled with your surgical or radiation oncologist. In some cases or after a period of time, you may choose to see your primary care provider for your on-going survivorship care. As you move further away from your treatment, your primary care provider will assume more aspects of your health care, so it is important to delineate clearly the roles of each of your medical providers. You and your healthcare providers should develop a care map and long-term surveillance calendar. A cancer summary should be generated that includes diagnosis and stage, cancer treatment received, frequency of follow-up visits and diagnostic studies, and a list of potential short-term and long-term side effects. It may be helpful to include your current medications and other health conditions as well.

Remember to periodically update your summary to reflect your current health status and medical care.

Your follow-up appointment schedule will depend on your type of cancer and your treatment, as well as your other health conditions. Oncologists will usually see cancer survivors every 3–4 months during the first 2 years after treatment, and then every 6 months for 2–3 more years before moving to a schedule of annual follow-up appointments. Many older cancer survivors will also need to see their primary care provider to monitor and manage their other medical problems. You may wish to speak with all of your healthcare providers about coordinating these visits.

At each visit, your oncology provider will decide whether or not you will need blood work, imaging studies, or procedures based on your type of cancer and its treatment or your symptoms at the time of your appointment. Some common tests include a complete blood count or metabolic profile, CAT scans or X-rays, or a colonoscopy or cystoscopy. These tests, studies, and procedures are performed to monitor for disease recurrence or development of long-term effects from your cancer treatment. Your primary provider or oncologist may also request screening tests for other cancers.

You may be cancer-free, but you may not be free of your cancer. Many cancer survivors continue to experience side effects from their disease and treatment even after they have completed therapy. Prompt evaluation of and intervention for the aftereffects of cancer and its treatments are imperative to maintaining your health, coping with the transition to wellness, and improving your quality of life.

MANAGING THE LONG-TERM SIDE EFFECTS OF CANCER AND ITS TREATMENT

Survivorship may come with a cost that impacts every domain of well-being—medical, physical, social, psychological, and economic. Older cancer survivors may be at a higher risk for a change in quality of life, since they often begin their cancer journey with underlying functional impairments and medical conditions or an age-related vulnerability that makes them more likely to experience short and long-term complications after completion of their treatment. The long-term and late effects of cancer treatment include cognitive changes, difficulty readjusting to life without cancer, onset of new or exacerbation of chronic medical conditions, and in some cases, premature death.

TREATMENT EFFECTS

Cancer and its treatments are associated with short and long-term complications. These adverse effects can be temporary or result in chronic health problems, and can be mild or life-threatening. Persistent effects that begin during treatment, like fatigue or chemotherapy-related neuropathy, can continue into survivorship. Late effects manifest after completion of therapy, and may undermine organ function and compensatory mechanisms necessary for successful living. Collectively, 75% of cancer survivors will experience some long-term effects, which may include:

- *Effects from your surgery.* Cosmetic changes such as removal of a breast or a colostomy may cause emotional distress and identity and sexual readjustment; lymphedema after axillary dissection may cause pain, swelling, and a decrease in function of the affected limb; there may also be functional changes related to amputation or loss of part or all of an organ (e.g., incontinence after prostatectomy or electrolyte derangements associated with a cystectomy) or chronic pain that may affect your quality of life and function.

- *Effects from radiation therapy.* Damage to skin can lead to skin cancer, and site-specific damage can lead to issues like dry mouth, dental decay, damage to heart and lung tissue, loss of bone density, cognitive impairments, incontinence, and risk for a second primary cancer such as thyroid or breast cancer or sarcoma.

- *Effects from systemic therapy.* Fatigue, persistent suppression of your blood counts, and stress are common. Other effects include kidney or bladder damage, hearing loss, heart damage, loss of or too much sensation, cognitive impairments, changes in how food tastes, or a second primary cancer such as leukemia. Chemotherapy or endocrine therapy for breast or prostate cancer may cause osteoporosis, weight gain, clotting abnormalities and heart disease, mood disturbance, and hot flashes.

Any or all cancer therapies can cause chronic health problems, functional losses, disruption in family life and role, caregiver stress, psychosocial distress, and collectively, diminished quality of life. Do not become frustrated if you experience these effects. You and your body need time to recover physically and emotionally from your treatment. Your medical providers will help you address these side effects and any new treatment effects that develop over time. For tips on coping with the long-term effects of treatment, please refer to http://www.cancer.gov, http://www.cancer care.org, and http://www.cancer.net.

LIVING A HEALTHIER LIFESTYLE

When you meet with your medical providers, it is important to develop a health promotion plan that may help you to take charge of your health and well-being, reduce your chances for a disease recurrence, or prevent a new cancer.

Health maintenance. Prior to your cancer, you may not have seen a doctor on a regular basis, or participated in a cancer or other health screening. Some older adults with severe health, functional, or memory problems may not benefit from cancer screening. Talk to your medical providers about whether or not cancer screening would be of benefit to you. Also, discuss recommended guidelines for prevention and treatment of heart and lung disease, hypertension, and diabetes.

Exercise. Recent studies suggest that staying active during and after your cancer care can help limit loss of function and the impact of long-term side effects, lower your risk for recurrence, and increase your long-term survival. Exercise also can reduce stress, fatigue, and pain; boost your immune system; and improve your mood, cardiovascular health, and sense of well-being. Before embarking on an exercise regimen, talk to your medical providers; they may recommend certain types of exercise to prevent injury or to account for your other health problems, such as heart disease or arthritis. Moderate exercise, like walking or swimming, at least 30 minutes a day, 3–5 times per week, is recommended. If you cannot exercise, deep breathing exercises, simple stretching, or change of position can prevent infections, skin breakdown, and loss of function and mobility.

Diet and nutrition. Eating a well-balanced diet and maintaining a healthy body weight is often difficult for older persons, but may help to reduce your risk of developing a new cancer or a recurrence of your cancer. Healthy eating also will promote cardiovascular health. Talk to your medical provider about any special dietary needs you might have as a result of your cancer and its treatment or your other health problems. Diets rich in green and orange fruits and vegetables, lean protein, and whole grains, and low in fat and salt are recommended. You can still enjoy rich and fattening foods, but remember the key to a successful diet is moderation!

Smoking cessation and limited alcohol consumption. Smoking, chewing tobacco, or exposing yourself to secondhand smoke can increase your risk of a new cancer or a recurrence of your cancer. Smoking also is bad for your heart and lungs. If you quit smoking during your treatment, congratulations and keep up the good work. If you have not quit, now is the time to try. Quitting is difficult so joining a support group, asking friends and family for support, or using anti-smoking medications such as a nicotine patch may help you to meet your goals. It may take several attempts before you can quit, but you can do it; after all, you just BEAT cancer! It also is a good idea to limit your alcohol intake since alcohol consumption has been shown to increase your risk for certain cancers.

Stress management. Cancer treatment and recovery, and life in general, are stressful! Worrying about your health, juggling your feelings and returning to "normal" can be overwhelming. Finding ways to reduce or control the stress in your life may help you to feel better and to cope with your recovery. Reducing stress also can improve your memory and mood, boost your immune system, and decrease your pain. Being well-informed about your cancer and what to expect in the future, expressing your feelings and being focused and optimistic, yet realistic, can help you to cope with your fears as you transition from treatment to surveillance. Activities such as exercise; meditation or relaxation; volunteer work; laughter; creative expression through art, hobbies, or keeping a journal; or participation in a support group also may help you to manage your stress and keep you focused.

Setting new and achievable goals. You have just completed a difficult journey and now are embarking on another journey called survivorship. Your life has likely changed in one way or another. You may see and feel things differently than before your diagnosis. Take some time to reassess your life and your goals. Ask yourself: What is important in my life? What do I want to do and how do I want to do it? What and who makes me happy? Talk with your family and friends and share your thoughts and experiences. Weigh your options and try new things.

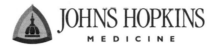

CHAPTER 7

PALLIATIVE AND COMFORT CARE

BY GRACE A. CORDTS, MD, MPH, MS

"Hope does not lie in a way out but in a way through."

—Robert Frost

Cancer and its treatment can cause various symptoms; this chapter will help you deal with these symptoms. These symptoms might include pain, nausea and vomiting, constipation, depression, anxiety, breathlessness (dyspnea), fatigue, delirium/confusion, and itching (pruritis). Your oncology team will talk with you about what symptoms you may experience as a result of your cancer and its treatment(s), and help you anticipate ways to deal with them before they become an issue.

Palliative care physicians specialize in taking care of symptoms. Many cancer treatment programs have palliative care physicians on their treatment team; your healthcare provider may ask that you see one to help with symptom management.

It is important to have good symptom management because it contributes to your well-being, allowing you to participate in life. For many older cancer patients, quality of life may be more important than longevity, and exactly how a symptom is treated will depend on the extent of your cancer and what goals you have for yourself.

This chapter also will discuss hospice and how hospice might help you and your family if your cancer treatment does not work, or if you decide you do not want to undergo any more anticancer treatment.

PAIN

You may already have experienced pain, or worry that you might have pain associated with your disease and its treatment. Uncontrolled pain not only causes physical discomfort, but also emotional, spiritual, and social distress. It can affect your appetite or sleep, and make you feel depressed, anxious, out of control, or like a burden. It is VERY important to let your doctor know if you are having pain. People sometimes worry that worsening pain means their cancer is getting worse. Although this may be true, it is not always the case.

At each office visit, your doctor will ask you a series of questions about your pain. You will be asked to rate your pain using a scale of 0–10 (0 being no pain at all and 10 being the worst pain ever experienced). Your doctor also will ask you to describe where the pain is, and whether it is a new or worsening pain. Other questions include: What does it feel like (sharp, throbbing, burning, cramping)? Is it intermittent or constant? How long has it been going on? What makes it better? What makes it worse? What have you used to treat your pain, including such things as over-the-counter medication like Tylenol (acetaminophen) and Advil (ibuprofen) or heating pad? How is the pain affecting your life? You might want to consider making notes about your pain that you can take with you to your next visit with your doctor.

Pain is treated with medications, as well as types of non-pharmacologic treatments; you may receive multiple types of treatment for your pain. Your course of therapy will depend on you and what works best for you. The nonpharmacologic ways to deal with pain include: physical therapy, exercise, acupuncture/acupressure, meditation, guided imagery, hypnosis, cognitive and behavioral therapies, relaxation, therapeutic massage, and support groups, to name just a few. All of these methods can be used in conjunction with your pain medications.

Pain also may be treated with more invasive procedures for local control of your pain. Your healthcare provider can help determine what is best for you and refer you to the most appropriate provider. If pain is coming from a specific place or nerve, a nerve block might help, which is similar to when you have Novocain (procaine) at the dentist's office. An anesthetic is injected around the nerve causing the pain, thus preventing the nerve from transmitting pain impulses. A physician with special training (usually an anesthesiologist or interventional radiologist) performs the nerve block. This physician can perform other pain-relieving procedures, such as placement of a catheter to give continuous pain or numbing medication or kyphoplasty, a special technique used to stabilize bone and reduce pain if you have a compression fracture in one of your vertebra.

Like nerve blocks, a short course of radiation therapy often provides excellent relief of localized pain. It is particularly effective in treating pain caused by cancer metastases to the bone; these localized therapies usually allow patients with cancer to lower or even eliminate their dose of narcotic pain relievers (opioids). Although these medicines do an excellent job of controlling pain, they often cause confusion, falls, and constipation in older patients.

The medications used to treat pain include over-the-counter medications like Tylenol and non-steroidal anti-inflammatory medications (NSAIDs), opioids, and other medications called adjuvant medications. Opioids such as morphine, oxycodone, methadone, dilaudid, and codeine are sometimes referred to as narcotics; in this chapter, the term opioids will be used. Adjuvant medications are medications originally developed for conditions besides pain, but have been found to help treat pain. These medications include antidepressants and antiseizure medications. How and when these medications are used are based on the World Health Organization's (WHO) three-step approach to cancer pain management based on the severity of your pain and the type of pain you are having.

If you have mild pain, over-the-counter medications like Tylenol and NSAIDs might be enough to treat your pain. You can take up to 3000–4000 milligrams of Tylenol a day, depending on your medical situation. Talk to your doctor about how much medication is right for you.

NSAIDs are medications that help with pain, especially if inflammation is involved. These are drugs like Motrin (ibuprofen), Advil, and Aleve (naproxen). You can get them over-the-counter at low doses or by prescription for higher doses. They are good for bone pain, but they can have significant side effects; if you have a history of stomach ulcers, gastritis, kidney disease, or liver disease, talk to your doctor before using them. Kidney function declines with age (see Chapter 5), and since NSAIDs can also reduce kidney function, older individuals should use them with caution and only with careful monitoring.

If these medications are not helping to control your pain, your doctor may suggest an opioid, which can be used with Tylenol or NSAIDs; there are some pain medications that are a combination of Tylenol or an NSAID and an opioid. If you are taking a pain medication that has Tylenol or an NSAID in it, you need to be careful about how much extra Tylenol or NSAID you take. Although the dose of an opioid can be increased, there is a limit to how much Tylenol and NSAID you can take before those medications may cause harm to you. Your doctor may suggest taking an opioid alone so that the opioid can be increased without causing toxicity from the Tylenol or NSAID.

Some people worry about becoming addicted to opioids. It is uncommon to become addicted to opioids, especially when you are taking opioids for pain associated with an illness. Talk to your healthcare provider if you are worried about this. If you currently have an addiction problem or a history of addiction, you need to tell your healthcare provider; this history is important since it will likely affect the amount of medication you need to control your pain.

There are a few terms to know that might help you understand the use and abuse of opioids: tolerance, physical dependence, and addiction (psychological dependence). Physical dependence is a normal physiological phenomenon that happens to everyone if they have been on opioids for a while. It refers to a withdrawal syndrome that occurs when an opioid is abruptly discontinued. Other drugs also can cause a physical dependence; for example, if you drink caffeinated coffee and stop drinking it and develop a head-ache, you are physically dependent on caffeine. This does not mean you have an addiction to caffeine. Tolerance is also a normal physiological phenomenon in which you need to increase the dose of the opioid to get the same de-gree of pain relief. Psychological dependence or addiction is a compulsive preoccupation with acquiring and using the medication for non-medical purposes, despite harm to the person.

The specific medication and dose that you take will depend on your situation. No two people are alike in their pain or what it will take to control it. One patient might need a much higher dose of medication than someone else. It will depend on how you metabolize the drug.

If you have pain all of the time, it is important to take some-thing regularly for your pain, whether it is Tylenol or an opioid. It is easier to manage your pain if you take some-thing before the pain becomes severe and the medicine has to "catch up" to the amount of pain you have. Many opioids have a long acting form such as MS Contin (mor-phine), Oxycontin (oxycodone), and Duragesic (fentanyl transdermal), so you do not have to take the medication as often. If your pain is constant, your doctor or healthcare provider will first use a short acting opioid to figure out how much pain medication you will need. You will take the short-acting opioid every 3 to 4 hours, and once your pain is controlled, a long-acting opioid, which you only have to take a couple of times each day, can be taken instead of the short-acting opioid; your healthcare provider also will give you short-acting opioids to take if you have more pain than usual. This additional pain is called breakthrough pain.

Sometimes pain can happen when you are doing a certain activity; this is called incident pain, and it is best to take a dose of your short-acting pain medication before starting the activity that causes your pain.

Opioids can be taken in different ways. Usually the medications are given orally in pill form; if you have trouble swallowing pills, some medications come in a dissolvable tablet (buccal form) or liquid form. Morphine comes in a concentrated liquid and a few drops can be taken orally, though it does not need to be swallowed. Most opioids can be given rectally, but not all. This route can be used temporarily, especially if it is during the night and you suddenly cannot swallow your pill or if you are using a pain pump and it stops working. However, if you have diarrhea, the rectal route is not an option. Long-acting opioids do not come in liquid or buccal formulations. If long-acting opioids are needed and you cannot take pills, a patch or an opioid pump may be prescribed for your pain control.

One opioid, fentanyl, comes in a transdermal formulation (Duragesic). The medication is in a patch that is applied to the skin and the medication is absorbed through your skin. There are a few instances when this formulation does not work well; if you are extremely thin or obese, the medication may not get into your system as well, or if the patch does not adhere to your skin because you have excessive sweating or skin rashes, then this delivery mode is not for you. There must be good contact between the skin and the patch for the transdermal fentanyl to work. Fentanyl also comes in a formulation that can be directly absorbed into the tissues of the mouth, though it can cause mouth irritation and should not be used if you have mouth sores. This is a short-acting medication and should only be used for breakthrough pain.

If you cannot take any oral medications, your opioid may be given through a small catheter subcutaneously or intravenously. The catheter is attached to a small pump and the opioid is delivered continuously (the basal rate), with extra (demand) doses for breakthrough pain intermittently. The intravenous route is usually only used in the hospital, but can also be used at home; you and/or your family will need to learn how to care for the catheter and pump if used at home. Medications can also be given through the epidural route. A catheter is placed in the spinal canal and pain medication is given through the catheter; an example of when this route is used is when a woman is giving birth to a baby and an epidural is given to control the pain.

Adjuvant medications are often used if you have neuropathic pain; this pain is usually described as burning, tingling, itching, or numbness. Adjuvant medications are usually used with opioids; some medications include Pamelor (nortriptyline), Cymbalta (duloxetine), Neurontin (gabapentin), Lyrica (pregabalin), Dilantin (phenytoin), and Tegretol (carbamazepine).

Corticosteroids, such as prednisone or Decadron (dexamethasone), also are used for the treatment of pain, especially pain due to swelling of the organs or spinal cord, or bone lesions. These medications help reduce inflammation. Corticosteroids also can improve your appetite and give you a sense of well-being. Corticosteroids are usually not used as a first-line treatment of pain because of the side effects they can cause, but they can be used initially if you are having pain from your cancer pressing on your spinal cord. Steroids are usually given for a short time. Corticosteroids do have a number of side effects that can be particularly problematic, and not uncommon, in older individuals, especially those who already have issues such as gastric irritation, depression, psychosis, fluid retention (that triggers congestive heart failure), or elevated blood sugar (diabetes). Muscle weakness (myopathy) and osteoporosis can also be a problem in those who take these medications for a long time. These side effects can usually be treated.

SIDE EFFECTS OF OPIOIDS

Opioids do have side effects. Some are more common than others, and several resolve after you have been on the medications for a few days. Common side effects include constipation, dry mouth, nausea/vomiting, and drowsiness. Uncommon side effects include hallucinations, delirium, itching, urinary retention, and muscle twitching.

CONSTIPATION

Constipation is a troublesome side effect, especially for older persons who may already suffer from chronic constipation, and it is a symptom that does not go away even after you have been on opioids for a while. You will need to take a stool softener and a laxative to prevent constipation. Unless your doctor tells you otherwise, you should start with two tablets of senna and two tablets of Colace (docusate sodium) twice a day. You also can add sorbitol, lactulose, or milk of magnesium as needed. The goal is to have a bowel movement every 1 to 3 days, or to maintain your normal stooling schedule. A new prescription medication, Relister (methylnaltrexone), is designed specifically for constipation from opioid use, and might be helpful if you do not have a bowel movement with the recommended bowel regimen. It is given subcutaneously, and it is important to stay near a bathroom after the injection, because it can work for some people in about 30 minutes; however, it can take up to 4 hours to see results. Enemas also can be used, and can be purchased at your local pharmacy or prepared at home using a very old homemade remedy of equal parts molasses and warm milk; however, a milk and molasses enema should not be used with children and infants. You may not be able to use an enema if your bowels are not intact, you have low white blood cell counts, or you have an active bowel infection. You should always talk with your healthcare provider before using an enema.

DROWSINESS

You may find yourself feeling drowsy after you take opioids, especially in the first few days after starting these medications. If someone has been in pain for a long time and finally has good pain relief, they can often sleep for an extended time; this should not be confused with drowsiness from the opioids. If the opioids continue to cause drowsiness, the dose can be reduced. If dose reduction does not work or you have more pain when the opioid is reduced, a stimulant like Ritalin (methylphenidate) might be helpful. Ask your doctor or healthcare provider about this.

NAUSEA

Nausea is a common side effect of opioids, as well as of cancer and its treatment. One option to treat nausea is to try another opioid; if this does not work, a medication can be used to control the nausea. These medications are called antiemetics. There are several different prescription medications that help with nausea: Kytril (granisetron), Zofran (ondansetron), Reglan (metaclopramide), Compazine (prochlorperazine), Decadron, Haldol (haloperidol), Ativan (lorazepam), or an antihistamine like Benadryl (diphenhydramine). There are several things you can do to help with nausea and vomiting, including:

- Eating smaller meals
- Avoiding foods with strong smells
- Eating bland food
- Eating food that is cold or at room temperature
- Avoiding greasy and high-fat foods
- Drinking ginger ale or sucking on peppermint candy
- Taking your medication with food
- Keeping your bowels moving

If your nausea and vomiting continues, talk to your health-care provider, as these symptoms may not be related to your opioid, but to something else.

PRURITIS

Itchy skin (pruritis) can be associated with opioids. The itching can be controlled with emollient creams, lotions containing aloe vera, anti-itch lotions (sarna lotion), and topical Benadryl cream. If this does not work, nonsedating antihistamines like Zyrtec (cetirizine), Allegra (fexofenadine), or Claritin (loratadine) may help. If you develop a rash or other allergic symptoms, tell your healthcare provider, as you may be allergic to the prescribed opioid.

MYOCLONUS

Muscle twitching (myoclonus) can occur when opioids are taken at high doses. The muscle twitching can be more concerning to your family members than you, though the twitching can interfere with your daily activities. If it does, ask your healthcare provider for help. Switching to another opioid, at a lower dose, can help to decrease or stop the twitching; if this does not work, a muscle relaxant may help.

CONFUSION

Delirium can occur in some people, especially older patients, with opioid therapy. A lower dose or a different opioid may clear up the confusion. Healthcare providers often start your opioid at a low dose and gradually increase the dose until you find the right amount that relieves your pain without causing confusion. Occasionally, you might hallucinate on opioids. The treatment for this is the same as for delirium: Change to another opioid or reduce the dose.

URINARY RETENTION

The inability to pass urine is an uncommon side effect of opioids, and is often the result of constipation from the opioid. The hard stool pushes against the urethra (the opening in the body from which urine drains), making it difficult for the urine to pass. When the constipation is treated, the urinary retention often resolves. In certain cases, the opioid itself can affect the bladder by making it impossible for the bladder to squeeze out the urine; this may be a problem for older men with enlarged prostates, and a reduction of the opioid dose usually resolves the issue. If a lower dose does not fix the problem, or the pain worsens on the lower dose, a Foley catheter may need to be placed into the bladder to allow the passage of urine. Urinary retention might not be related to your opioid, but rather your other medications, or your disease or its treatment. If you develop new urinary symptoms, remember to tell your healthcare provider about it.

OTHER SYMPTOM MANAGEMENT

DYSPNEA

Shortness of breath (dyspnea) is a common symptom found in people who have cancer. It can be scary to be, and

94

scary for your family to see you, short of breath. This symptom may be related to your cancer or its treatment, or other conditions such as emphysema, congestive heart failure, pulmonary embolus (blood clot in your lung), or anemia. If you have new shortness of breath, your doctor might want you to get some tests—a chest X-ray or CAT scan, PFTs, blood work, or an echocardiogram—to see what is causing the problem. If a specific cause of your dyspnea is found, your healthcare provider might suggest a specific treatment. If fluid around your lung (an effusion) is causing your shortness of breath, a needle can be used to drain off the fluid. If your cancer is pushing on your lungs or airway, radiation therapy might be helpful. Nebulizer treatments, inhaled medications, or steroids can help open up constricted or inflamed airways. If you have a low oxygen level, oxygen therapy may help you feel better. Having a fan in the room, which circulates a breeze across your face, also can help. A change in your position, such as propping yourself up on pillows, also may make you feel better. Breathing exercises can help with shortness of breath, but in order to be helpful, these exercises need to be learned and practiced before you suffer an acute case of dyspnea. If you feel a little short of breath, breathing in through your nose and out through your mouth may help. If you have persistent shortness of breath, low doses of opioids have been shown to be an effective treatment. Some healthcare providers and patients are reluctant to use opioids for this purpose because of concerns that the opioid will make you stop breathing, but this has not been the case when opioids are used appropriately. If you or your medical provider has these concerns, try a low dose of medication when someone will be with you.

Some people may experience severe or sudden shortness of breath at the end of life. If you have a disease or cancer that may cause severe shortness of breath, it is important to plan ahead on how to cope with and treat it. When you are acutely short of breath and in crisis, it is difficult to make a plan. Ask your healthcare provider to help you come up with this plan, which might include going to an inpatient hospice unit for symptom management or the use of opioids and inhaled treatments.

ANXIETY

Anxiety is more than just worrying. There is a lot to think about when you are sick, but anxiety is worry that interferes with you enjoying yourself or thinking clearly. It is what keeps you up at night, with your mind racing. Some people also may experience physical symptoms like palpitations, sweating, sleeplessness, or dyspnea. Anti-anxiety medications and talk therapy can help control your anxiety. Benzodiazepines are anti-anxiety medications used to treat debilitating anxiety; these medications include Ativan, Valium (diazepam), Klonopin (clonazepam), and Xanax (alprazolam). Some antidepressants also can help with anxiety.

DEPRESSION

Depression is a condition that is common in older persons, and it can also occur when you have cancer. It is common to feel sad when you are given a diagnosis of cancer or if your disease is progressing or not responding to treatment, and people often say it is normal to be depressed in this situation; however, while it is normal to be sad, being sad is different from depression. If you have no interest in activities or find no happiness in what you once enjoyed, you might be suffering from clinical depression. Other signs of depression include feelings of worthlessness and hopelessness, and thoughts that others would be better off without you. Some symptoms that are associated with depression, like a change in appetite or sleep, or fatigue, may be related your disease and are not good indicators of depression. It is important that you or your family tell your healthcare provider if you are feeling depressed, so that you can be diagnosed and treated promptly. It is important to seek treatment for depression since it can have a major impact on your quality of life.

Take care in choosing an appropriate antidepressant, since many of these agents, including tricyclics and monoamine oxidase inhibitors (MAOIs), aggravate a number of medical problems that are common in older individuals, including: urinary retention related to an enlarged prostate, constipation, blurred vision, low blood pressure, rapid heart rate, and cognitive impairment. Often, selective serotonin reuptake inhibitors (SSRIs) are preferred, as the side effects are less troubling in older persons.

NAUSEA AND VOMITING

Nausea and vomiting are not only caused by opioids, but also by many other conditions, including your cancer and its treatment, electrolyte imbalances, irritation of the stomach, and constipation. Dehydration is common in older people, and nausea and vomiting can make it worse. The same suggestions outlined earlier for nausea/vomiting associated with opioids can be of use here. Your healthcare provider will try to figure out what is causing the nausea and vomiting and then treat the underlying cause. If constipation is causing the problem, resolving the constipation with an enema, suppository, or medication will help. If you have gastritis, a drug to treat that could be helpful.

CONSTIPATION

Constipation is a common symptom of people with cancer, even if you are not on an opioid. It is easier to prevent constipation than to treat it. Older people often already suffer from constipation because of being on multiple medications, age-related slowing of the gastrointestinal tract, and being less active. If you are on an opioid, you should always be on a bowel regimen that promotes a bowel movement daily, or every other day, unless there is a specific reason not to be on one. There are several things *you* can do to help promote bowel movements: drink plenty of water, get some exercise, and be sure that you have fiber in your diet.

FATIGUE

Fatigue (tiredness) is a common symptom in patients with cancer. Fatigue can be from stress, chronic medical conditions, the treatment of other health problems or cancer, or from the cancer itself. If medication is causing fatigue, you can try to decrease its dose or switch to a different one. Insomnia can add to fatigue; getting adequate amounts of sleep may be difficult with cancer, but behavioral treatment has been shown to be the most effective treatment of insomnia. Techniques include: having a sleep schedule and nightly routine; avoiding caffeine, alcohol, and nicotine; having a light snack before bed; not drinking any fluids for several hours before bedtime; using your bed for sleep only (not for other activities such as reading or watching TV); and trying to get exercise during the day. You may have more energy during certain times of the day; if this is the case, try to plan activities around that time of day. Ask family and friends to help with chores that need to be done. If none of this helps and the fatigue is interfering with what you want to do, a brief trial of a medication like Ativan,

Ambien (zolpidem), trazodone, or melatonin may be used to "reset" your sleep patterns, or a stimulant like Ritalin may be prescribed to keep you more alert and active.

DELIRIUM

Confusion (delirium) can be a distressing symptom for you and your family to deal with. Delirium can occur as a result of certain medications; fatigue; changes in environment, hearing, or vision; infection; urinary or bowel retention; or immobility. Older patients may be more likely to experience delirium as a result of chronic health problems, multiple medications, and underlying cognitive problems; as such, it is a VERY common symptom during acute hospitalization and at the very end of life. It impacts your ability to communicate with your family and your medical team. There are several simple things that you can do to decrease your risk of becoming delirious, including surrounding yourself with familiar items like family pictures, using your eyeglasses and hearing aid, trying not to nap during the day, moving around as much as you can, staying organized, and trying to keep things stress-free and calm. Your doctor will work with you to figure out what is causing this confusion and make changes in your care to decrease it, if possible. If these things do not help, your doctor might give you medications called antipsychotics like Haldol or Risperdal (risperidone), which have been shown to help with delirium.

HOSPICE CARE

Often, when people think about hospice, they think of a place; in fact, hospice refers both to a philosophy of care and a Medicare benefit. Patients are said to receive hospice care when the goals of treatment focus on comfort rather than cure. The Medicare hospice benefit, discussed here, is well-defined medical care for people who are at the end of their life; many other insurance companies provide a hospice benefit.

The goal of the Medicare hospice benefit is to improve quality of life for people with a terminal diagnosis and their families, by supporting them through the last few months of life. The hospice team provides a multidisciplinary approach to symptom management with medical, nursing, psycho-social, volunteer, and pastoral care services; also, they provide bereavement services for families for up to 13 months after the death of their loved one. Hospice services can be delivered in a patient's home, a nursing home, assisted living facilities, or at an inpatient hospice facility. In the United States, most hospice services are provided at home, with the family providing the hands-on care. Inpatient hospice is usually provided only when someone has acute symptoms that cannot be controlled at home or is imminently dying.

These services are provided by all certified Medicare and Medicaid hospices, and hospices may offer additional services with the money they raise through donations. For you to be eligible for the Medicare benefit, you must be enrolled in Medicare, have an estimated life expectancy of 6 months or less, and no longer be receiving curative therapy for your cancer. You must be able to receive most of your care at home and have a caregiver who will assume the responsibility for your physical care if you are unable to care for yourself. You should identify a decision maker in the event you cannot make decisions. Many hospices are now providing services that are palliative, like radiation or chemotherapy, which they traditionally have not covered. If you are not quite ready for hospice, there are bridging services provided by some hospices that are associated with home health agencies; they provide services while you are receiving active treatment. For these to be paid for by Medicare, you must have a skilled need and be homebound; however, you do not need to be homebound to receive hospice services.

CONCLUSION

Although the symptoms and side effects of cancer and its treatment can be overwhelming, there are ways to make you feel better. Do not hesitate to talk with your healthcare providers about your symptoms and concerns; if they do not know about them, they cannot help you.

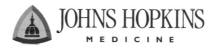

CHAPTER 8

THE VALUE OF PLANNING AHEAD

BY LESLIE PIET, RN, MA, CCM

When confronted with a diagnosis of cancer, patients experience a cascade of emotions and mentally live through the possible outcomes associated with their disease and its treatment. After the initial roller coaster ride, patients hope for the best possible outcome—cure and long-term survival—but also need to plan ahead in case the best outcome is not their reality. Planning ahead will help you and your loved ones meet some of your personal, emotional, spiritual, and physical needs.*

Whether you are of an older age, or have cancer or another life-threatening disease, advance planning is important to consider not only for you, but also for your family. This chapter will review some of the issues that you might want

* Note that any recommendations or resources listed are only suggestions, not endorsements.

to discuss with your family and healthcare providers; in this case, family members may include children, spouses, partners, parents, siblings, nieces or nephews, cousins, and close friends.

Talking to your friends and family about your values and concerns can help put your mind at ease. Prior to the onset of an illness, you may not have thought about or taken the time to discuss this topic; it is important to talk about these issues with your friends and family in order to open up a dialogue about end-of-life preferences and goals of treatment. Patients want their wishes respected and concerns addressed, and caring family members want to be equipped to help and support their loved ones. If advance care planning is overwhelming to you, consider involving a spouse or other trusted family member, a close friend, your doctor, a social worker, or an elder lawyer, legal aid, or other attorney to help you process your thoughts and start the conversation.

TALKING WITH ADULT CHILDREN OR OTHER FAMILY MEMBERS

If you have just been diagnosed with or have been living with cancer, you are faced with the "what ifs" associated with your disease and treatment: What if I get sick and cannot take care for myself? What if my treatment does not work? Your family is also very concerned about what might happen to you and is thinking about how they can help you manage your illness. Although it is sometimes a difficult task, taking the time to talk with your family about the multiple possible scenarios is very important. For example, if you have an aged spouse for whom you are the primary caregiver and are worried about what will happen if you are too sick to care for him or her, share your concerns with your family. This information will help them to address your needs and coordinate care for you and your spouse. If you find it difficult to start the conversation, you might want to ask your healthcare provider, social worker, or clergy to help you think about what you want to say and how to say it.

ADULT CHILDREN TALKING WITH AN ILL PARENT OR RELATIVE

Some adult children are not sure how to approach an elderly parent or relative they are concerned about, fearing that talking about topics related to dying will upset him or her. This conversation should be held in a relaxed environment and discussed tactfully and according to the desires and energy level of the patient involved. Sometimes, a family conference with a social worker can be of great value in beginning the process of talking about sensitive issues.

Asking your parent if and when it would be okay to discuss the subject of advance care planning is another approach that can be used. Remember, the conversation is meant to teach you about your parent's healthcare and personal wishes so that you and others can respectfully carry them out. Once you have had a conversation about your parent's healthcare preferences in the event of a life-threatening illness or event, it is important to document this discussion so that other members of your family, your parent's friends, and your parent's healthcare providers can abide by his or her treatment goals and instructions for medical decision making.

ADVANCE DIRECTIVES (LIVING WILLS)

The Patient Self-Determination Act of 1990 requires Medicare and Medicaid providers to offer adults who are being admitted to healthcare agencies such as hospitals, nursing facilities, home health, and hospice the opportunity to complete or submit their advance directives (ADs). An AD is a written or oral opportunity to describe what you do or do not want for your health care if you are faced with a life-threatening illness and cannot speak for yourself. An oral AD may be completed when a patient talks with a healthcare provider and a note about the conversation is written into the patient's record; a written AD is portable and readily available in case a person is taken to a hospital or care facility where the patient record is unavailable. Local healthcare agencies can educate you about ADs and the state policies regarding them. It is voluntary to complete an AD, and agencies cannot discriminate against a person who decides not to complete an AD. However, an AD gives you an upfront opportunity to participate in making healthcare decisions. Items that may be included in ADs are:

1. Designation of a healthcare agent (durable power of attorney for health care [HPOA])

2. Direction regarding life-support treatment

3. Instruction for emergency situations

4. Organ or body donation instructions

Each state in the United States has an AD document. There are other documents, including the Five Wishes document, that can be found at your local hospitals, lawyers' office, or on the internet.

HEALTHCARE AGENT (HEALTHCARE POWER OF ATTORNEY)

When completing the AD, you also may appoint a person to speak for you if you cannot speak for yourself, and to determine the course of your health care within the terms documented in your AD. This person may be called a healthcare agent, medical decision maker, healthcare power of attorney (HPOA), or another title. Remember, state laws may vary; if you travel from one state to another (to visit family or during different seasons), it may be especially important to have a document that also complies with laws in those other states.

In the second part of the AD, you can state your preferences for the events associated with a life-threatening illness or end-stage condition. An AD gives you the opportunity to clearly state your values and goals of care. You can state your wishes as absolutes (yes or no), or gradations of care (e.g., brief trials of a lifesaving intervention). You can state what you don't want done, and more importantly, *what you do want done.*

Remember, *no AD document can cover all situations.* Writing down your goals and wishes can help your HPOA make decisions based on your best interests. Remember, if you change your mind in the future, you can always change your AD.

When you complete an AD, it is very important to make sure that you discuss your AD with your medical providers and your HPOA and that they have a copy of your written AD. Keep a copy for yourself in a place where it can be easily retrieved in case of an emergency or if you need to go to the hospital.

WHAT CAN HAPPEN WITHOUT AN ADVANCE DIRECTIVE?

Memories of past conversations with loved ones about your wishes may become very fuzzy under the stress of an acute or life-threatening illness. Unless doctors know your wishes, they may do procedures, administer treatments, and use machines that you do not want. This could happen even if your chances of surviving the event or living with your disease may be very poor. Well-meaning family members may pressure your loved one to do more tests and procedures that may have limited benefit. Your wishes may not be carried out if they are not clearly known.

Not clearly spelling out your wishes invites conflict. Convictions on what to do may waver under pressure from well-meaning healthcare providers or family members. Having what you want in writing may help decrease family conflict and guilt.

HOW TO TALK ABOUT AN ADVANCE DIRECTIVE: AN AD PARTY

It is often uncomfortable to talk about your potential death, even though we all know death is inevitable. Even if we do not have firsthand experience with deathbed situations, the media has brought them into our homes and hearts; in response, many of us have said, "I don't want to die like that." ADs may be the answer. As previously discussed, talking about your treatment wishes and goals is often easier said than done. Some have found it helpful to jump-start the process by holding an Advance Directive Party, where family and friends gather together to discuss their end-of-life wishes and complete their ADs. The AD party creates a comfortable environment in which to address uncomfortable, yet important, topics. The Five Wishes document (with its educational DVD) can be used to facilitate the process. In most states, it will serve as your AD; other states require that it be attached to a state-approved AD document. Be sure that the document that you choose for your AD complies with your state laws and regulations. If you want more information about the Five Wishes document, go to http://www.agingwithdignity.org/five-wishes.php.

DO NOT RESUSCITATE/DO NOT INTUBATE FORMS

Emergency medical technicians (EMTs) typically do not have time to read your AD in an emergent situation; instead, the EMT will often look for a do not resuscitate (DNR) or do not intubate (DNI) form that is completed by your provider based on the goals expressed in your AD. These forms allow the EMTs (who take patients to the hospitals in ambulances) to provide comfort care measures to patients who do not desire aggressive management, such as cardiopulmonary resuscitation (CPR) and intubation. If you have a life-threatening illness, it is helpful to have a DNR/DNI form along with your AD. You should also post a copy of the DNR/DNI form on your refrigerator or next to your telephone, so if a caregiver calls 911, the DNR/DNI form may help to ensure that your wishes are honored by the EMT personnel. Some state laws provide for individuals to wear DNR/DNI bracelets. Talk with your healthcare provider about the type of forms and procedures used in your state.

PHYSICIAN ORDERS FOR LIFE-SUSTAINING TREATMENT

The Physician Orders for Life-Sustaining Treatment (POLST) form is used in some states for patients with a life-threatening illness. Unlike an advance directive, the POLST is a medical order signed by a physician. The orders expressed in a POLST should support what the patient indicated in his or her advance directive. Exact forms and policies can vary by state. Some similar forms are referred to as MOLST, MOST, or POST forms. All are intended to formalize patient treatment decisions with medical orders that can follow the patient when transferred from one health facility to another. More information can be found at http://www.polst.org.

OTHER IMPORTANT ISSUES TO ADDRESS AS YOU PLAN AHEAD

Just as you have planned ahead for medical decision making scenarios associated with a potentially life-threatening or no longer treatable illness, you also should consider how to address your nonmedical affairs, including your finances, will, funeral, and personal and business relationships.

DURABLE POWER OF ATTORNEY (POA) FOR FINANCES

The role of a POA for finances is *very different* from the role of a healthcare agent. The POA for finances helps the patient take care of money-related matters, like management of bank accounts or payment of bills. It does not cover healthcare-related issues. For that, you will need a separate HPOA. Your local bank or your attorney can help you with the process of appointing a POA for finances.

WILLS

A will is a legal document in which you state how you would like your personal property and goods distributed after your death. Unlike the POA for finance and the HPOA, a will does not provide for your financial or healthcare-related needs while you are still alive. An attorney can be a valuable resource for helping you to complete your will; other resources include your local office on aging, retired senior volunteer programs, or the local register of wills.

In addition to having an up-to-date will, you should make sure that all of your affairs are in order. Make certain that your personal papers are well-organized, up-to-date, and in one place so that a trusted friend or family member can access them if needed. You also may want to give a copy of all your important papers to your lawyer. Do not forget to include information about your insurance policy and beneficiaries, checking and savings accounts, stocks, bonds, retirement accounts, safety deposit boxes, property titles, and car titles. You may want to consider having a predesignated beneficiary or cosigner on your checking, savings, and investment accounts. Your attorney can advise you regarding these and other matters pertaining to your estate planning.

Registering a Will

Many counties have a local register of wills that, for a small fee, will keep a copy of your will on file for safe-keeping. They also can help open up estates, get letters of administration, and give general advice (for legal advice, you must consult a lawyer). You should also make sure that a family member, friend, or lawyer knows where you have a copy of your will and where it is registered.

What Could Happen Without a Will

The estate of someone who dies without a will is subject to local laws. Some states will give 50% of the estate to the surviving spouse and 50% to the minor children; inheritance rules for stepchildren may be different than for biological children. If the person does not have any living children, the estate may be divided between the spouse and the deceased's parents. If the spouse of the deceased is the only one alive and there are no other heirs, the spouse may be the only recipient. If there are no living heirs, the money could go to some place like the local department of mental health or Board of Education. If you are concerned about where your money and property will go after you are gone, consider drafting a will. Be sure to update your will as your life circumstances change. A thoughtfully written and frequently updated will that expresses clearly your wishes on how you would like your estate and personal belongings distributed can minimize family conflicts that may arise if there is no will. Remember that outstanding bills and debts may be paid from the estate.

FUNERAL PLANNING

Although it is often difficult to think about your funeral, there are several questions that you may want to discuss with your family or friends. Have you already purchased a cemetery plot? Have you made financial or other arrangements with a particular funeral home? Where do you want to be buried? Do you want to be cremated? Do you want a funeral service?

Funeral Costs

Funeral services can be expensive. Some counties have specific laws regarding burial; your funeral director can tell you what they are and how much they cost. Funeral homes and crematoriums are required to provide price lists, which you can use if you decide to purchase additional services.

If your financial means are limited, the funeral director or a social worker may direct you to services that might help to defray the cost of burial. Some places of worship and organizations also may offer assistance with burial costs, and a person who received medical assistance may be eligible for a small amount of money from the state towards funeral expenses. Social Security provides a one-time benefit of about $250 when a person dies; someone will need to notify Social Security that you have died and follow their process for receipt of this benefit. You can find more information at http://www.ssa.gov.

Veterans

Veterans, spouses, and dependent children are eligible to be buried under the Veteran's Death Benefit; an honorable discharge form, the DD214, is needed for eligibility of this benefit. If you cannot locate this form, seek help from your social worker, the Veteran's Administration, or go to the Web site http://www.va.gov; you can also call (800) 827-1000 for further information. Consider contacting an American Legion or VFW post, as they may have dedicated personnel to help veterans and families with paperwork associated with funerals.

If you have the DD214, you will need to present it to the funeral director who will help coordinate activities between the funeral home and the military cemetery. They will also help obtain a United States flag to drape the coffin of the veteran. The 21-gun salute, the flag folding over the coffin, and the military funeral are incredible to behold in honoring the veteran who has honorably served his/her country.

REFLECTING ON RELATIONSHIPS

There is a book titled *The Four Things That Matter Most: A Book About Living,* by Dr. Ira Byock, a palliative care doctor and specialist in end-of-life care and medical ethics. This book tells stories about relationships and offers reflections on what we should say every day to those we care about, but which often become more important when we are faced with a life-threatening illness. The four most important things to say are:

1. Please forgive me.

2. I forgive you.

3. Thank you.

4. I love you.

Completing the Four Things helps with relationship closure and healing. Those who are able to complete their unfinished business in relationships are often at greater peace. You may want or need to say some or all of the Four Things. Forgiveness tends to be the most universal thing; it resonates with most people and is applicable to many personal and business relationships. We have all experienced the regret associated with a lost opportunity to express our love, respect, and concern to a family member or friend. Consider taking the time to say the Four Things to your family and to others. Taking responsibility for your behavior and sharing your feelings with your loved ones can open up a door for others to send some of that love and forgiveness back to you.

We plan for many things in life, but do not always plan for issues involving life's end. Consider doing some advance planning based on your beliefs, values, and goals.

Having a plan will allow you and your family to cope with the changes in your health and address your end-of-life needs. Talk openly with family, friends, and healthcare providers. Share with them your fears, hopes, and wishes for the present, future, and end-of-life. Discuss your treatment preferences and healthcare goals. Seek legal counsel as needed. Address personal and financial matters in a timely manner, and organize your important documents. Reflect on what is important to you! And remember that planning ahead is a loving act for your family and for you!

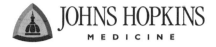

CHAPTER 9

PHYSICAL MEDICINE AND REHABILITATION

BY RICHARD D. ZOROWITZ, MD

The loss of function from cancer and its treatment can significantly impact the quality of life of all patients. In older patients, there may be a greater burden of preexisting functional impairment, which may result in additional limitations in activity as compared to younger patients. Addressing functional issues comprehensively can prevent further decline during treatment of your cancer, and may help to restore you to a premorbid state of function and total well-being.

Rehabilitation, otherwise known as physical medicine and rehabilitation (PM&R) or physiatry, is a branch of medicine that emphasizes the prevention, diagnosis, and treatment of disorders related to the nerves, muscles, and bones that produce temporary or permanent deficit(s) in function. Physiatrists often are acknowledged as functional or quality-of-life physicians because of their ability to address issues that help a patient to be more physically and functionally independent. Older cancer patients may require the services of PM&R physicians, physical therapists, occupational therapists, or speech-language pathologists, as their baseline function may be impacted by sequelae of their cancer or other health problems, or side effects from treatment. Rehabilitation medicine provides integrated and holistic care in an attempt to retrain a patient to his maximal physical, psychological, social, work, and recreational potential. Addressing these issues must take into account the symptoms with which the patient presents at time of consultation, such as weakness, numbness, or speech problems, and those that occur during or after cancer treatment. The living situation of the patient, use of devices to make activities of daily living easier (e.g., cane, walker, commode, tub seat), driving issues, or work issues also may need to be addressed to facilitate treatment and improve function.

TYPES OF REHABILITATION CARE

To understand rehabilitation care, one must be able to describe human function. The World Health Organization devised the International Classification of Function, which organizes all aspects of human health and well-being. In this classification scheme, *body functions* are the physiological and psychological functions of body systems. *Body structures* are anatomical parts of the body, such as organs, limbs, and their components. *Impairments* are problems in body function or structure (e.g., muscle weakness, numbness, speech problems). *Activity* is the execution of a task or action by an individual (e.g., walking, bathing, dressing, grooming). *Participation* is involvement in a life situation (e.g., working, driving). *Activity limitations* are difficulties an individual may have in executing activities. *Participation restrictions* are problems an individual may experience in involvement in life situations. *Environmental factors* make up the physical, social, and attitudinal environment in which people live and conduct their lives. PM&R practitioners will use this terminology to assess your functional health, and define interventions specific to your personal and functional needs.

Many problems caused by cancer can be addressed by rehabilitation medicine. These include physical and cognitive impairments, pain, tissue swelling, and psychological disturbances. Deconditioning, neurologic disorders, and disruption of lymphatic flow are common underlying etiologies of these problems. Patients with cancer can benefit from treatment utilizing well-established rehabilitation techniques within an interdisciplinary framework; however, rehabilitation may be more complicated because of the wide range of functional issues that occur during a patient's oncologic diagnosis and treatment. For example, radiation or chemotherapy may help to shrink the size of a tumor, but at the same time, these treatments also may cause fatigue that affects a patient's ability to function adequately.

Rehabilitation care includes preventive measures directed toward reducing impairments or activity limitations that may arise from your chronic medical conditions or your cancer and its treatment. For example, patients hospitalized for long periods of time can easily become deconditioned, which may be prevented by mobilizing the patient through an appropriate exercise program, even during the procedure and recovery period!

Restorative rehabilitation aims toward re-establishing a patient's level of function to a level better than or similar to one prior to the patient's illness. For example, patients who develop proximal muscle weakness after receiving high doses of corticosteroids can benefit from early therapeutic exercise and mobilization.

Supportive rehabilitation maximizes the function of the patient with new long-term impairments or activity limitations, such as training a patient with weakness in a leg to walk, or weakness in an arm to feed, dress, bathe and groom his- or herself.

Palliative rehabilitation provides comfort and support to patients with advanced or end-state disease, and their families, by decreasing a patient's dependence on others for mobility and performing activities of daily living. By decreasing the amount of assistance required for a patient's transfer from bed to chair or commode, home care may become a more viable option for caregivers and may lead to an improved quality of life for the patient and his or her caregivers!

ORGANIZATION OF THE REHABILITATION TEAM

The rehabilitation team consists of many professionals who contribute their individual skills to improve the overall condition of the patient. As the team is patient-centered, the patient must be able to state goals of care with respect to impairments, activities, and participation in the proposed treatment. Each team member is responsible for contributing to a patient's care using his or her own expertise, as well as for monitoring issues that can be conveyed to and addressed by other team members, including your oncologist and primary care provider. This open communication facilitates the execution of the treatment plan and optimizes functional outcomes.

An *interdisciplinary team model* allows team members to work within their own sphere of expertise but act in coordination with other team members and patients to set and coordinate functional goals. Team conferences are used to report functional progress, make decisions as a group, and develop an optimal patient care plan. The patient becomes the center of the team and plays a significant role in the goal setting required for transition back to his or her baseline function. There is an active exchange of ideas that might alter the types of therapy given to a patient as new goals or plans emerge.

Like the interdisciplinary team model, the *transdisciplinary team model* encourages communication among healthcare professionals, but also encourages cross-treatment among disciplines. The transdisciplinary team model is based upon the premise that the team members with the expertise and understanding of certain functions can work more efficiently and effectively on the same goals. Cross-training allows better patient evaluations, goal setting, and treatments. For example, both physical therapists and occupational therapists may train a patient in walking; the physical therapist may train the patient to walk a certain distance, but the occupational therapist may train the patient to walk in a kitchen to perform a cooking task. The transdisciplinary team allows its members to work on common patient-determined goals so that all members have an opportunity to work on all aspects of function, rather than their own exclusive areas of expertise. This allows patients to work longer and more intensively on areas of mobility and self-care, and attain better outcomes in a shorter period of time. The transdisciplinary team model is well-suited for the care of older patients with cancer.

MEMBERS OF YOUR REHABILITATION TEAM

While your primary care physician or oncologist coordinates your overall medical care, referral to rehabilitation care means that you will be served by a coordinated team of professionals that complement your general medical and cancer treatment(s). The rehabilitation team may be composed of some or all of the professionals described in this section.

- *PM&R physician.* The physiatrist usually coordinates the rehabilitation team and manages medical conditions related to a patient's cancer diagnosis and his/her chronic health conditions. A physiatrist is a physician specializing in PM&R, and physiatry focuses on the restoration of function to patients with problems ranging from decreased mobility to complex cognitive or functional complications. Physiatrists may provide rehabilitation care to patients with a variety of neuromuscular or musculoskeletal conditions, such as muscle weakness, numbness, speech problems, or cognitive problems. These problems can be exacerbated by your cancer and its treatment; for example, some chemotherapy drugs can cause neurologic symptoms such as numbness, or aggravate a preexisting neuropathy.

- *Rehabilitation nurses* (http://www.rehabnurse.org). Rehabilitation nurses manage complex medical issues, collaborate with other specialists, provide ongoing patient and caregiver education, and establish plans of care to maintain optimal wellness. Rehabilitation nurses take a holistic approach to meeting patients' medical, work-related, educational, environmental, and spiritual needs. Rehabilitation nurses act not only as caregivers, but also as coordinators, collaborators, counselors, and case managers in both the inpatient and outpatient environments.

- *Physical therapists* (http://www.apta.org). Physical therapists are experts in the examination and treatment of neuromuscular and musculoskeletal problems, such as muscle weakness or coordination, that affect patients' abilities to move. Through exercise training and management, physical therapists help to enhance joint, muscle, heart, and lung function. They use a number of modalities, including heat, cold, electrical stimulation, and compression therapies to treat complications caused by cancer or its treatment. Physical therapists also direct treatment towards preventing injury and loss of movement, and they work in many inpatient and outpatient settings.

- *Occupational therapists* (http://www.aota.org). Occupational therapists help patients achieve independence in all facets of their lives. They give patients the skills necessary for independent and satisfying lives. Services that occupational therapists typically provide include customized treatment programs to improve one's ability to perform daily activities, comprehensive home and job site evaluations with adaptation recommendations, performance skills assessments and treatment, adaptive equipment recommendations and training, lymphedema treatment to reduce swelling in the limbs, and education to family members and caregivers. Although there are overlaps in the functions of physical and occupational therapists, occupational therapists are more involved in retraining of hand and arm functions, while physical therapists tend to be more involved in problems of leg and trunk functions.

• *Speech-language pathologists* (http://www.asha.org). Speech pathologists assess and treat language and speech disorders such as aphasia (problems with language), speech apraxia (inability to perform learned muscle movements needed for speech), dysarthria (slurred speech), and cognitive-communication disorder (inability to transform thoughts into meaningful speech). They also treat people with swallowing disorders that may result from surgery, radiation treatment, or chemotherapy. This type of therapy is particularly important in older head and neck cancer patients who may have a harder time adapting to swallowing and other functional disabilities that follow operative and chemo-radiation treatments. Many of these patients go to nursing homes for several weeks after treatment, and often do not get adequate rehabilitation and swallowing therapy.

• *Neuropsychologists* (http://www.apa.org). Neuropsychologists specialize in studying brain–behavior relationships and have extensive training in the anatomy, physiology, and pathology of the nervous system. They may diagnose and treat problems with memory, attention, and other issues with thinking. Some cancer patients may experience changes in their memory or experience confusion as a result of their chemotherapy treatments, surgery, or radiation to the brain; the issues may be new, or treatment procedures may unmask or aggravate chronic cognitive problems. A neuropsychologist might use tests to identify and treat cognitive and neurobehavioral dysfunction, as well as monitor the course of recovery and the patient's potential for return to the baseline function. Neuropsychologists also may help to diagnose and treat mood disorders such as depression or anxiety.

- *Recreational therapists* (http://www.atra-tr.org). Recreational therapists are specialists who utilize various activities as a form of active treatment to promote the independent physical, cognitive, emotional, and social functioning of persons disabled as a result of trauma or disease; this is accomplished by enhancing current skills and facilitating the establishment of new skills for daily living and community functioning. In addition, recreational therapists assist the patient in developing social skills, discretionary time skills, decision-making skills, coping abilities, self-advocacy, discharge planning for re-integration to home and community, and skills to enhance general quality of life. Many recreational activities may promote wellness among cancer patients coping with their disease and social re-integration among patients with brain tumors or peripheral nerve problems caused by chemotherapy. Patients may also be seen by a horticultural therapist (http://www.ahta.org), music therapist (http://www. musictherapy.org), dance therapist (http://www.adta. org), art therapist (http://www.arttherapy.org), or animal-assisted therapist (http://www.deltasociety.org).

- *Social workers* (http://www.naswdc.org.) Social workers assist individuals to restore or enhance their capacity for social functioning, while creating societal conditions favorable to their goals. Social workers help patients and their families overcome the effects of poverty, discrimination, abuse, addiction, physical illness, divorce, personal loss, unemployment, educational problems, disability, and mental illness. They help prevent crises and counsel individuals, families, and communities to cope more effectively with the stresses and stressors of everyday life and life with cancer. Social workers identify resources that allow patients with disabilities to remain in the community, and if the patient cannot live in the community, the social worker helps them apply for medical and financial assistance, and also identifies short-term and extended-care facilities.

- *Certified rehabilitation counselor* (http://www.crccertification.org). Rehabilitation counseling is a systematic process that assists patients in the community with physical, mental, developmental, cognitive, and emotional disabilities to maximize their work and leisure-time goals.

- *Prosthetists and orthotists* (http://www.abcop.org). Prosthetists and orthotists make and fit braces and splints (orthoses) for patients who need added support for body parts that have been weakened by injury, disease, or disorders of the nerves, muscles, or bones. They work under a physician's orders to either adapt purchased braces or create custom-designs. Orthotics are often named for the body part(s) they cross, such as AFO (ankle-foot orthosis) or KAFO (knee-ankle-foot orthosis). Orthotics such as Halo braces (a brace that surrounds the head and is held in place with small screws in the skull) or TLSO (thoracolumbar spinal orthosis) may be used to stabilize portions of the spine and prevent further damage to the spinal cord after injury. A prosthetist makes and fits artificial limbs or prostheses for patients with disabilities. These include artificial legs and arms for patients who have had amputations due to conditions such as cancer, diabetes, or injury.

- *Other professionals.* A variety of other specialists may be part of your rehabilitation team. An oncologist, surgeon, or neurosurgeon may consult on the patient to treat specific cancers. The patient may require other medical or surgical specialists to monitor new or chronic health conditions throughout the course of rehabilitation. A psychiatrist may be asked to manage the emotional aspects of cancer and its treatment. Podiatrists (http://www.apma.org) address foot health problems, especially in patients with diabetes, peripheral vascular disease, or peripheral neuropathies. Peripheral neuropathies are common in cancer patients, both from chronic medical conditions or their cancer and its treatment. A dentist (http://www.ada.org) cares for teeth or dentures, especially in patients with head and neck cancer. They also address regimens for oral hygiene and dental side effects associated with cancer treatments (e.g., mucositis, mouth sores, loosening of teeth, and bone loss in the jaw). Less commonly, prosthetics such as palatal lifts may be necessary to close the soft palate and permit more normal swallowing function. An audiologist (http://www.asha.org) evaluates your hearing and works with patients who require hearing and speech rehabilitation. They also fit and dispense hearing aids and other assistive devices. Since certain tumors and chemotherapy may affect your hearing, audiologists can help to ensure that you can improve your ability to hear or participate in your daily activities despite a hearing loss.

Cancer and its treatment can cause a wide variety of functional problems, including difficulties with walking, self-care, language, cognition, swallowing, and pain. Rehabilitation professionals help your oncology team determine if you are fit enough to tolerate the rigors of cancer treatment, and if not, they may be able to devise a plan to get you there. Their treatments are designed to improve or maintain your performance before, during, and after cancer therapy.

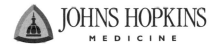

CHAPTER 10

PHARMACY: CHEMOTHERAPY, SIDE EFFECTS, AND DRUG INTERACTIONS

BY BRYNA DELMAN EWACHIW, PHARMD

A s discussed in Chapter 4, treatment of your cancer may include surgery, radiation therapy, chemotherapy, or any combination of the three. Chemotherapy can be in the form of oral or intravenous antineoplastic medications, immune modulator therapy, hormonal therapy, or oral or intravenous targeted therapies. Your oncologist will determine which chemotherapy regimen is appropriate for you and your cancer type. The aging process (see Chapter 5) can affect the activity of many chemotherapy agents, both oral and intravenous, that are prescribed for your cancer treatment. As patients age, their ability to break down (metabolize) and remove (excrete) many types of medications, including chemotherapy, is sometimes diminished. In some instances, elderly patients may experience more side effects than younger patients.

Your oncology provider may need to reduce or modify your chemotherapy doses if you have changes in your kidney, liver, or heart function. Chemotherapy also is affected by changes in body composition, such as hydration status, muscle-to-fat ratio, nutritional status, and your overall health. Your cardiovascular, neurology, and immune functions, which often change as you age, may affect how well you will tolerate your chemotherapy.

Age alone is not a predictor of how a patient will tolerate a specific treatment. Since aging is an individualized process, every patient tolerates chemotherapy and its side effects differently. Your healthcare providers will perform a global assessment of your health and well-being and use their findings to prescribe an appropriate and individualized regimen for treating your cancer (see Chapter 4). Your providers will reassess your global health and cancer status throughout your treatment course in order to minimize side effects and maximize benefit. Side effects from chemotherapy, radiation, and surgery can range from mild to severe. Your healthcare team will review with you common side effects that you may experience from your treatment. It is important to inform your healthcare providers about any side effects that you are experiencing from your treatment, and you should notify them immediately if your side effects persist or worsen.

SIDE EFFECTS

Some common side effects caused by chemotherapy include nausea, vomiting, diarrhea, constipation, pain, hair loss, and skin reactions. Your providers will prescribe medications before, during, and after your treatment to minimize or prevent these side effects. It is very important that you take these medications as prescribed. Most patients will receive medications, such as Zofran, Kytril, or Anzamet (dolasetron), with or without a steroid such as Decadron, to prevent nausea and vomiting. You may require additional medications to treat delayed nausea and vomiting after your chemotherapy or radiation treatments. Chemotherapy can also cause changes in your liver, heart, or kidney function (see Chapter 5).

KIDNEY

Kidney function declines as we age. Some of the medicines that older patients take to treat both their cancer and non-cancer-related problems might make this worse. The dehydration that often accompanies cancer and its treatment can put additional stress on the kidneys. Fortunately, it is often possible to minimize these effects by carefully selecting and dosing appropriate drugs, managing potential adverse drug interactions, and preventing dehydration.

COGNITIVE EFFECTS

Neurotoxicity and cognitive effects, also known as chemo brain, can be profoundly debilitating in patients who are already cognitively impaired. Elderly patients with a history of falling, hearing loss, or nerve damage have decreased energy and are highly vulnerable to neurotoxic chemotherapy like the taxanes or platinum compounds. Many of the medicines used to control nausea (antiemetics) or decrease the side effects of certain chemotherapeutic agents are also potential neurotoxins; these include Decadron (causing psychosis and agitation), Zantac (ranitidine; causing agitation), Benadryl, and some of the antiemetics (causing sedation).

HEART

Heart problems increase with age, and it is no surprise that older cancer patients have an increased risk of cardiac complications (especially congestive heart failure) from anthracyclines and other potentially cardiotoxic anti-cancer agents. Patients treated with Platinol-AQ chemotherapy require large amounts of intravenous fluid hydration, which can cause congestive heart failure in patients with heart problems; these patients should be monitored carefully.

BONE MARROW

Anemia (low red blood cell count) is common in the elderly, especially the frail elderly. It decreases the effectiveness of chemotherapy, and often causes fatigue, falls, cognitive decline, and heart problems; it is essential that anemia be recognized and corrected with red blood cell transfusions or the appropriate use of erythropoiesis-stimulating agents like Procrit and Epogen (epoetin) or Aranesp (darbepoetin).

Myelosuppression is also common in older patients getting chemotherapy or radiation therapy. Older patients with myelosuppression develop life-threatening infections more often than younger patients, and they may need to be treated in the hospital for many days. The liberal use of granulopoietic growth factors (such as G-CSF, Neupogen [filgrastim], and Neulasta [pegfilgrastim]) decreases the risk of infection, and makes it possible for older men and women to receive full doses of potentially curable chemotherapy.

Thrombocytopenia, or low platelet cell count in the blood, can cause serious bleeding problems; this is especially worrisome in an older person who is prone to falling. Someone who bleeds into the brain can suffer a serious and debilitating stroke. Like anemia and myelosuppression, thrombocytopenia is a side effect of many chemotherapy medicines, especially Paraplatin (carboplatin), and radiation therapy. It can usually be successfully managed by checking blood counts frequently and transfusing platelets when appropriate.

DIARRHEA

Diarrhea is another common side effect of certain chemotherapy agents such as Camptosar (irinotecan), Adrucil (fluorouracil), and Eloxatin (oxaliplatin). Patients treated for colon and/or rectal cancer often experience diarrhea from chemotherapy and/or radiation treatments. Many over-the-counter agents are available for the treatment of diarrhea (such as Imodium AD and Pepto-Bismol [bismuth subsalicylate]), as well as some prescription remedies (Lomotil [atropine and diphenoxylate], Sandostatin [octreotide]). Dehydration is not uncommon in older people, and untreated diarrhea can aggravate this to a point where hospitalization is required. Infections, other medication, and bowel obstruction can also cause diarrhea, so talk with your provider before taking any agents to treat your symptoms.

MUCOSITIS, NAUSEA, AND VOMITING

Like diarrhea, mucositis, nausea, and vomiting can cause severe dehydration in older patients who often are already dehydrated due to inadequate fluid intake and use of diuretics (or water pills, usually prescribed to treat high blood pressure or heart failure). Careful monitoring and the liberal use of rehydration drinks (like Pedialyte) and intravenous fluids are essential components of the management of older cancer patients, especially those receiving radiation, 5-fluorouracil (5-FU), or both.

PAIN

Pain is a common symptom among patients with cancer. It may be directly related to your cancer or a side effect from your cancer treatment. Your provider may prescribe pain medications to manage your pain. Your provider and nurse will ask you to describe where your pain is and what it feels like, and they will also ask you to rate your pain each time you visit the clinic. Your providers may prescribe either narcotic or non-narcotic medications to manage your pain. Non-narcotic pain relievers include Tylenol, siacylates, or NSAIDs, and can be purchased over the counter. Some non-narcotic pain relievers can affect your kidneys or liver, or interfere with your platelet function, so talk with your provider before taking any non-prescribed pain medications. Many narcotic pain relievers (oxycodone, morphine, or hydromorphone) can cause constipation. Your providers will give you medications to manage constipation, and most of these medications are over-the-counter (Colace, senna, or Milk of Magnesia) and can be purchased in many drug stores/supermarkets. Elderly patients also can experience constipation from changes in their diet, inactivity, other chronic medical conditions, surgery, or chemotherapy.

OSTEOPOROSIS

Loss of bone density can be made worse by AIs, which are the most common form of hormonal therapy in post-menopausal women with breast cancer. This, in turn, can result in fractures, falls, and progressive debility. All older women should have a DEXA scan before starting an AI, and if you are not already doing so, you should take appropriate calcium and vitamin D supplements. If you have been taking these supplements regularly, and your bone density scan shows significant osteopenia or osteoporosis, you should start taking oral bisphosphonates such as Fosamax (alendronate sodium), Actonel (risedronate sodium), or Boniva (ibandronate sodium). If you only have osteopenia, and have not been taking calcium and vitamin D, it is reasonable to try these supplements first. By following your bone density on repeated DEXA scans, your doctor can see if these oral therapies are working. Most insurance companies will pay for only one DEXA scan a year; this is usually enough in this situation.

If these measures do not work, intravenous bisphosphonates, such as Zometa (zoledronic acid) may allow you to remain on an AI. Another possibility is that, if you have no major risk factors like blood clots, your doctor may consider switching to Soltamox (tamoxifen). It is still an excellent drug for both early stage and advanced breast cancer, and it has less risk of aggravating osteoporosis. Women who are prone to falling, or have already had a broken bone due to osteoporosis, should probably avoid the AIs all together.

Men receiving androgen deprivation hormonal therapy for their prostate cancer can also have problems with osteoporosis. Older men on hormonal therapy should have regular DEXA scans to monitor their bone health and, when appropriate, take calcium and vitamin D supplements or bisphosphonates to minimize bone loss.

POLYPHARMACY

Cancer treatments can be complex, and patients and their caregivers often have to manage appointments, lab tests, scans, and numerous prescriptions. Older patients often have chronic illnesses that can also impact their cancer care, and they may take prescription and over-the-counter medications for their chronic conditions that can interact with certain chemotherapy treatments. Upon your first visit to the cancer center, it is important to bring with you a current list of all your prescription and over-the-counter medications and supplements. You may want to bring the actual medications to your appointment so that a nurse or pharmacist can accurately obtain a detailed medication history and review it for possible redundancy and drug–drug and drug–disease interactions. The nurse and pharmacist will also need to obtain your allergy history. Your medication history will be reviewed with you each time you visit the cancer clinic or upon admission to the hospital. It is a good idea to carry in your wallet an index card with a list of your allergies and all of your current medications, including your chemotherapy regimen.

When patients have multiple health conditions, are seen by multiple healthcare providers, and fill their prescriptions at multiple pharmacies, they are at increased risk for polypharmacy. Polypharmacy means "many drugs." It occurs when you take more than five medications, and it puts you at risk for adverse drug events, overlapping side effects, and drug–drug interactions. People taking multiple medications, especially older individuals, are more likely to confuse medicines, doses or schedules. Though most common in the elderly population, polypharmacy also affects the general population. Some of your medications may interact with each other or your chemotherapy agents. Your oncologist may need to adjust or change some of your non-cancer-related medications if they interact with or increase the likelihood of significant side effect from your chemotherapy. These adverse events can be prevented by using one pharmacy for all of your prescription needs, keeping a current medication list, and communicating with your pharmacist and provider(s) about new prescribed or over-the-counter medications and supplements.

An example of a medication that might interact with your chemotherapy is Coumadin, a medicine prescribed to thin your blood. Your oncologist may need to adjust your Coumadin regimen or you may require more frequent blood draws to monitor your INR, a lab test to determine whether or not your Coumadin is at a therapeutic dose. The oncologist may ask you to stop taking aspirin, or NSAIDs like Advil, or Aleve, all of which can also interact with chemotherapy or affect your platelets. Tylenol is a safe alternative for mild to moderate pain, as it does not interact with chemotherapy or your platelets. Other medications that may interact with your chemotherapy include antibiotics or cholesterol-lowering agents. Medications prescribed for your high blood pressure or diabetes may also need to be adjusted while on chemotherapy.

The use of complimentary or alternative therapies is common among cancer patients. Most natural or homeopathic medications are NOT approved or monitored by the Food and Drug Administration. Although these products may be "natural," they do have side effects and can interact with your chemotherapy and other medications. The Memorial Sloan-Kettering Cancer Center's Integrative Medicine Service Web site (http://www.mskcc.org/mskcc/html/11570.cfm) provides evidence-based information about herbs, botanicals, and supplements.

It is important to check with your oncologist before taking *any* medication or supplement not prescribed by your oncologist or primary care provider.

PAYING FOR YOUR MEDICINE

The cost of your cancer care, including laboratory and imaging tests, appointment copays, medications for your other health problems, and chemotherapy and its supportive medications, may sometimes pose limitations to your ability to adhere to your prescribed regimen. If you cannot afford some or all of your medications, please talk to your healthcare provider. Many pharmacies offer inexpensive generic medications, such as antibiotics and antinausea medicine, and a 90-day supply by mail order may be a less-expensive option for medications that you take for long periods of time. All patients older than 62 years of age may be eligible for Medicare programs for health care; Medicare Part A covers hospital admissions and Medicare Part B pays for outpatient treatments, tests, and most chemotherapy agents. Medicare Part B may also cover supplies and home healthcare services. Medicare Part D is a voluntary prescription plan that requires an annual enrollment, and there are many Medicare Part D prescription plans available. It is advisable that all patients enroll in a prescription benefit plan early in their treatment course to avoid out-of-pocket (uncovered) expenses. Part D programs vary by cost, coverage type, and the drugs covered. You and your caregivers should select a Part D program that best suits your medication needs; your pharmacist and social worker can provide more information about prescription coverage and Part D programs. You may also be eligible for other medication assistance programs funded by pharmaceutical companies or different social and charitable organizations. Your social worker can review these options with you.

FOLLOWING YOUR DOCTOR'S ADVICE

As patients begin their chemotherapy treatment, it is very important to follow the instructions given by the oncologist and the cancer center staff. Taking all of your medications on schedule and as prescribed can positively impact your cancer care. This is called *adherence to medical advice*. Some tips for staying adherent are to: (1) use a pill box or medication timers; (2) develop a routine (e.g., take your twice daily medicines when you brush your teeth in the morning and at night); and (3) keep a detailed diary of your medications, when you take them, and what side effects, if any, that you experience. Older patients often experience changes in their short-term and long-term memory that may lead to nonadherence to their medications. Having friends or family present during appointments may help you to remember the information provided about your illness and treatment. Older patients often experience a loss of hearing and changes in their vision, which may lead to difficulty following instructions and reading medication labels. Instructions for medications and other medical information in large print may be helpful for older patients. Pain or deformity from arthritis or numbness of one's fingers might impair an older patient's ability to open a medication vial or pick up a pill. Remember to request pill bottles that are easy to open or ask someone to help you fill a pill box.

When you are diagnosed with cancer, you and your caregivers will have a lot of questions about treatment options, types of chemotherapy available, and what types of side effects you could experience. There are many resources available to you and your caregivers. You will receive a handbook about your cancer and information about your chemotherapy regimen when you visit the cancer center. It is very helpful to have a spouse, family member, or friend accompany you during your first appointment, first treatment, and follow-up visits.

There are additional resources available to you and your caregivers through ACS and the NCI, as well as disease-specific organizations such as the Susan B. Komen Foundation and the Leukemia and Lymphoma Society. There is a wealth of information on the Internet about your diagnosis and treatments, though you need to careful about visiting only reputable sites; your cancer center staff might suggest Web sites that provide easy-to-understand, accurate, and up-to-date information about your medications/treatments, such as http://www.medlineplus.gov, http://www.chemocare.com, and others referenced in Chapter 12.

Your oncologist and cancer team, including nurses, pharmacists and social workers, will be available to answer all of your questions and provide you with assistance in coordinating all aspects of your cancer care. They are your best resource, and will help you and your family to navigate effectively through your treatment!

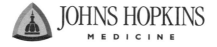

CHAPTER 11

NUTRITION IN THE GERIATRIC ONCOLOGY PATIENT

BY SWETHA MANOHAR, RD, LDN

M any cancer patients experience a loss of appetite (anorexia) and weight and a decrease in their energy due to their cancer and its treatment. Older cancer patients may be at a greater risk for these symptoms because of coexistent illnesses, poor or no dentition, social isolation, lack of access to food or its preparation, multiple medications, and a limited budget. The amount of weight loss varies with your type and stage of cancer, the treatment(s) you receive, and your other health conditions; however, if you have lost more than 10% of your weight in a period of 6 months or less, you are at an increased risk for nutritional deficits, decreased physical function, diminished quality of life, poorer response to your cancer therapy, and shortened survival. If you have lost weight, have a decreased appetite, or have barriers to proper food intake at the time of your diagnosis or at any time during your therapy, your oncology provider might request that you have a consultation with a nutritionist or a dietician, someone who specializes in the science of nutrition and in formulating diets to meet the special nutritional needs of patients with cancer and other illnesses. The goals of nutritional support include maintenance of or improvement in your function, quality of life, muscle mass, nutritious food intake, and total weight.

NUTRITIONAL ASSESSMENT

In order to assess your nutritional needs, your oncology provider and nutritionist will perform a thorough physical exam and take a detailed history. They will ask you questions about your weight 5 years, 1 year, and 6 months ago to understand how much weight you have lost or gained and how quickly you have lost or gained it. They will ask you about your favorite foods, changes in your appetite and ability to taste foods, and problems with swallowing or digesting your food. A review of your symptoms will focus on nausea, vomiting, diarrhea, constipation, indigestion, bloating, dry mouth, mouth sores, fatigue, weakness, and changes in urination. Your provider may draw a blood sample to assess your albumin, blood counts, kidney and liver function, blood sugar, and iron and nutrient levels. Each assessment will be based on your presentation, cancer, treatment, and individual needs.

IMPACT OF CANCER ON YOUR NUTRITIONAL STATUS

Cancer itself can cause you to lose weight, muscle, and your appetite. Your change in nutritional status is dependent on your baseline nutritional health, current symptoms, and cancer type and stage. Some cancers, such as pancreatic cancer, are associated with significant weight loss, while other cancers may induce little to no weight loss. Advanced cancers or cancers that cause inflammation are often associated with unexpected weight loss due to shifts in your metabolism, and may lead to loss of lean body mass, muscle, and fat. Loss of lean body mass, or cachexia, can lead to decreased functional capacity and diminished quality of life. Mechanical obstruction from your tumor may interfere with your ability to swallow, digest, or absorb your food, or you may feel bloated or full after eating only a small amount of food. Pain or nausea with food intake may act as a negative reinforcement for feeding even after the pain has resolved.

Treatment of your cancer also may interfere with your ability to maintain your weight. Surgery may alter the structures or integrity of the organs needed for chewing, swallowing, and digesting your food. In the postoperative period, you may experience nausea and your bowels might be sluggish. Inflammation from your surgery may cause you to lose your appetite or to have diarrhea. Radiation therapy may cause inflammation of your esophagus, stomach, or bowels, which may interfere with your ability to eat, taste, swallow, digest, and process your food. Chemotherapy may be associated with fatigue, nausea, diarrhea or constipation, mouth sores, a change in your taste sensation, and indigestion. All or any of these can lead to decreased food intake, inadequate hydration, and weight loss. Loss of weight can affect your energy level, sense of well-being, and even your ability to tolerate or benefit from the treatment for your cancer. Thus, maintaining your energy stores and weight by way of an adequate and proper diet is a very important part of your cancer care and treatment plan.

NUTRITIONAL INTERVENTIONS

A nutritionist will review your weight loss history and current diet and calorie intake, calculate your body mass index (how your weight relates to your height), take an inventory of your current symptoms, and assess your energy needs based on your activities. She or he will generate a palatable and nutritious diet to maintain or increase your weight during your illness and treatment. Your proposed diet will focus on whole foods instead of those that are highly processed, so that you may derive the maximum benefit from the food's healing properties, such as vitamins, minerals, amino acids, and phytochemicals. Your diet may change as your symptoms or treatment changes.

The nutritionist also may provide you with some tips on how to maintain overall health and a good nutritional state, including proper food handling and preparation; sharing and preparing meals with friends and family so that you may enjoy your meals and feel encouraged to eat; keeping convenience foods within reach around the house; eating more when you feel well; and maintaining good oral health—frequent tooth brushing and flossing and ensuring proper denture fittings. Foods with antioxidative properties, such as fresh fruits and vegetables, are highly recommended to help fight off free radicals in the body. Adequate hydration is encouraged. Sources of liquid in your diet can include water, juice, noncaffeinated and noncarbonated beverages, nutritional supplements, soups, ices and sherbets, and water-rich foods like melon and grapes. Although intensive exercise is not recommended during treatment, keeping physically active is encouraged as it helps stimulate your appetite and keep you energized.

Good nutritional health is important to your overall well-being, and it also may help with the management of side effects experienced during chemotherapy and/or radiation.

NUTRITION AND SYMPTOM MANAGEMENT

NAUSEA AND VOMITING

Nausea is a side effect of cancer that can occur from treatment, the stress of the cancer itself, constipation, or pain. Nausea can involve dry heaving and sometimes can lead to vomiting. Because food occasionally exacerbates the onset of these side effects, many patients tend to decrease their intake of food and fluids. If you decrease your overall intake, this could lead to further dehydration and a loss of energy; dehydration also can make you nauseous, which restarts the cycle.

There are several ways to manage your nausea. If nausea is brought on by chemotherapy or radiation, patients are prescribed antiemetic medications to help prevent nausea and vomiting. For these medications to be effective, it is crucial to take them at the time specified by your physician. Taking an antiemetic or a motility agent as needed before meals to prevent nausea may allow for optimal nutritional intake during mealtime. A proton pump inhibitor or an H2-blocker may also be prescribed to control nausea resulting from inflammation of the esophagus or stomach acid build-up. Nontreatment-related nausea and vomiting can be managed by stress-relieving exercises, meditation, and diet. The following nutrition tips may help you to eat or drink more when you are experiencing nausea and vomiting:

- Eat small, frequent meals throughout the day.
- Enjoy your meal—eat slowly and chew your food well prior to swallowing.

- Base your diet on bland, easily digested foods like cooked rice and vegetables, mild broths, dry toast, and applesauce.

- Avoid foods with strong odors and tastes.

- Chew on some ginger root or sip some ginger tea.

- Drink plenty of fluids, especially if you have episodes of vomiting and your intake of solid food is minimal. This is essential, as being dehydrated could make the nausea worse.

- Sit at a 45° angle during mealtime and try to avoid lying down for up to 2 hours after you have finished your meal.

- Choose a relaxed and peaceful environment in which to enjoy your meals.

- Share a meal with friends or family whenever possible.

MOUTH PROBLEMS AND CHANGES IN TASTE

During chemotherapy or radiation, changes in the taste or smell of foods, a sore or dry mouth, and irritation of your esophagus can occur. Chemotherapy medications may be excreted in your saliva, often imparting a metallic taste. It also may alter your taste buds, and the texture and consistency of your food may feel different in your mouth. Foods you may have liked in the past may no longer be palatable, and the palatability of food may change with each treatment or even from day to day. Many patients lose their "sweet tooth."

To address your change in taste, it is important to maintain good oral health and hygiene. Brushing your teeth regularly, flossing, and making use of mouthwashes, especially prior to meals, can help cleanse and refresh your palate. Performing periodic taste tests may be helpful for identifying palatable foods—use sugar for sweet, lemon for sour, salt for salty, and tonic water for bitter. Soft and fatty foods may taste better because they require less chewing, and thus, less saliva production. Supplements such as zinc (to counter sweet aversion) and B-vitamins may help minimize your changes in taste. In most cases, your taste sensation will come back once your therapy has ended. In the meantime, to help with taste alterations, try the following:

- Use plastic silverware if you experience a metallic taste in your mouth.

- Marinate foods with citric flavors such as lemon, but avoid this if you have sores in your mouth because the acidity might irritate them.

- Dress up your food with sauces such as barbecue or light soy sauce.

- Bring out the flavors of food by using fresh herbs, onions, and garlic to season foods.

- Sprinkle your food with brown sugar to alleviate bitter tastes in the mouth.

- Try easy-to-digest protein-rich foods like peanut butter, tofu, chicken, or fish.

- Chew on gum or suck on hard candy or mints.

To help with a sore/dry mouth:

- Focus on softer foods, such as soups, yogurt, cereals with milk, macaroni and cheese, puddings, and scrambled eggs.

- Add moistness to food with gravies or sauces.

- If you can tolerate it, try cold foods like popsicles, frozen fruits, and smoothies. If not, stick to room temperature foods and avoid very hot or cold food.

- Soak dry foods like cookies or bread in milk or another liquid.

- Avoid acidic foods like citrus fruits and tomatoes, as well as pickled and spicy foods.

Sometimes, if you are receiving radiation therapy to the head and neck or chest, you may experience a sore throat, find it difficult to swallow, or experience gastric reflux. If this is the case, follow the preceding instructions, but also try eating small meals, avoiding spicy foods, taking your time to eat, and thickening your foods. To thicken foods, try adding gelatin, tapioca, commercial thickeners, or cornstarch. Be sure to sit up during meals and for at least 2 hours after eating. If you consistently feel like you are choking or cannot swallow, consult your oncology provider immediately.

CONSTIPATION

An absence of regular bowel movements is another potential side effect of cancer and its treatment. There are several nutrition tips that can be used to help relieve constipation, in addition to the bowel regimen that your medical provider may prescribe. A gradual increase in your overall fiber intake will help stimulate and regulate the bowel, but it is important to remember that as you increase your fiber intake, you also will need to increase your fluid intake to at least 8 cups daily; otherwise your constipation may get worse. To ensure that you are drinking enough fluids each day, you can supplement your liquids with foods with a high water content, such as spinach, watermelon, soup, and Italian ices. To help manage constipation, try the following:

- Choose fresh fruits and vegetables.

- Include whole grain foods such as sprouted, whole wheat, rye, oat, or bran breads and cereals.

- Try other types of grains, such as quinoa, triticale, and kamut.

- Add dried beans and nuts to both cooked and un-cooked foods.

- Try brown or wild rice, as opposed to white rice, for some added fiber.

- Choose a high-fiber snack like a cereal bar (with 4 g of fiber or more per serving), dried prunes, blackberries, or wheat crackers.

DIARRHEA

Diarrhea, frequent bowel movements that are not formed, may occur as a result of a bowel obstruction, radiation or chemotherapy, noncancer related medications, or treatment of an infection with antibiotics. When you have diarrhea, you also may experience nausea, abdominal cramping and pain, fatigue, and dehydration. Water and nutrients are lost in the stool, and it is VERY important to drink fluids to match the fluid lost with your diarrhea. To help with intake of foods and liquids, try the following tips:

- Avoid products that contain lactose if it exacerbates your diarrhea.

- Try yogurt with active cultures to restore your healthy gut flora.

- After each loose stool, drink a few ounces of an oral rehydration solution such as Pedialyte.

- Limit the intake of high-fat and high-sugar foods, as this may worsen your diarrhea. This includes foods such as gravies, butter, sausage, fried meats and vegetables, colas, and drinks containing high fructose corn syrup. Instead try lean meats, steamed or boiled vegetables, and unsweetened beverages.

- Limit sugar-free foods made with sorbitol.

- Try to avoid spicy foods.

- Limit high amounts of fiber in the diet. Focus more on cooked vegetables and fruits, such as canned soft fruits that are packed in water, not syrup.

- Eat small meals throughout the day.

- Follow a B-R-A-T diet: bananas, rice, applesauce, and toast.

If you have more than three watery stools per day, or if you have bloody diarrhea, run a fever, or have abdominal pain, contact your healthcare provider immediately.

DECREASED APPETITE

You may experience a decrease in your appetite as a direct result of your chronic health problems, medications, and your cancer and its treatment, or as an indirect result of emotional stress and fatigue. If you have a poor appetite, try the following:

- Make large batches of food and freeze them, so that they are easily accessible later.

- Keep nonperishable foods such as cereal bars, applesauce, canned fruits, and peanut butter around the house.

- Drink beverages after you are finished with your meal, as drinking during meals may fill you up faster.

- Eat and drink more when you are feeling well.

- Try nutritional supplements such as Boost or Ensure between meals to add calories and protein to your diet. Mix milk, ice cream or yogurt, and peanut butter, fresh fruits, or juice in a blender for an instant energy-filled milkshake or smoothie!

- Experiment with new foods, textures, and tastes.

- Eat high-calorie, high-protein foods as snacks or meals—peanut butter sandwiches or crackers, nuts, macaroni and cheese, milk (including soy milk and yogurt), or eggs are just a few of the options.

- Eat with a companion.

Many of the side effects of cancer and its treatment make meal preparation and eating a less than pleasurable experience. If you live alone, have little appetite, experience fatigue or weakness, or do not have transportation, the procurement of food and the preparation of nutritious, well-balanced, and satisfying meals may be difficult and tiring. Do not be afraid to ask for help from friends and family. Be creative and try new foods by sampling prepared dishes from your local supermarket. Ask your grocery store if they have a shopping service that will deliver the food to you, or consider Meals on Wheels. Your nutritionist will help you come up with a diet to meet your needs. For a sample diet/menu, see Table 1.

If you cannot maintain your nutrition with a well-balanced diet, you may require nutritional support by other means. Patients who are unable to swallow, digest, or absorb their

Table 1 Sample Menu

Breakfast	2 hard-boiled eggs
	1 cup of oatmeal
	½ cup of fresh fruit
	1 cup of soymilk/milk
AM Snack	1 granola bar
	1 small piece of fresh fruit
Lunch	Tuna fish sandwich on whole grain bread
	Mediterranean salad (mixed greens, olives, feta cheese, tomatoes, carrots)
	Yogurt and fruit smoothie
PM Snack	Peanut butter and crackers
Dinner	Grilled chicken breasts with an herb sauce
	Steamed mixed vegetables
	Mashed potatoes with gravy
	Chocolate pudding
	Unsweetened iced tea

Fluids: Water throughout the day. Limit caffeinated and carbonated beverages.
Consult your dietician for a more personalized menu based on the side effects you may be experiencing and your caloric and protein needs.

food cannot maintain their weight, lean body mass, and well-being by eating a healthy diet. When patients are unable to meet their nutritional needs by eating readily available foods, feeding may be accomplished by either intravenous (parenteral) or tube (enteral) feedings. Intravenous feedings may occur through a catheter placed in your arm or into a central vein in your neck or chest. Feeding by catheter is called peripheral or total parenteral nutrition. Feeding by a tube placed either in the stomach or small intestine is called enteral nutrition. Feeding formulas are made up of carbohydrates, protein, fat, vitamins, and minerals and deliver nutrition directly to your body without you needing to take food in orally. These techniques are often used to maintain nutrition and weight during radiation therapy of the head or neck, esophagus, or stomach, or in patients with a mechanical obstruction. If an alternative method of feeding is prescribed, tube feeding is preferred when possible since it is more likely to maintain the integrity and function of the bowel lining, maintain your healthy gut bacteria, and enhance immune function. Parenteral nutrition is often necessary if a patient has a fistula, severe inflammation of the bowel, or a high-output bowel obstruction. If a feeding tube is recommended, your medical team, together with a dietician, will help you with the placement and care of your tube, formula selection, and timing of feeds. You will be transitioned back to an oral diet whenever possible.

FOOD SAFETY GUIDELINES

In addition to helping you maintain your weight, a nutritionist also will provide you with tips on how to handle food products safely to help eliminate contamination and reduce the risk of infection. Some basic tips include:

- Clean work surfaces in the kitchen with soap and water.

- Wash hands prior to preparing food or eating, and when switching between vegetables and meats.

- Wash hands with soap and warm water, or non-comediogenic gel soaps such as Cetaphil.

- Discard leftovers older than 2 days, unless frozen.

- Wash all raw fruits and vegetables prior to cooking or consumption.

- Cook raw meat to an internal temperature to at least 185° Fahrenheit.

- Thaw foods in the refrigerator.

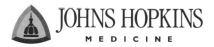

CHAPTER 12

TRUSTED RESOURCES—FINDING ADDITIONAL INFORMATION ABOUT CANCER AND ITS TREATMENT IN OLDER ADULTS

CANCER INFORMATION AND SUPPORT

A number of nonprofit organizations provide educational materials on a variety of cancer topics, including specific cancer types, various cancer treatments, and cancer research programs, to help you and your family make informed decisions about your care. Many also offer support services for anyone affected by cancer. Some cancer specific programs include the following.

American Cancer Society (ACS)
(800) ACS-2345 (227-2345)
http://www.cancer.org

CancerCare
(800) 813-HOPE (813-4673)
http://www.cancercare.org

Cancer.Net

(888) 651-3038

http://www.cancer.net

The Leukemia & Lymphoma Society

(800) 955-4572

http://www.lls.org

National Cancer Institute

(800) 4-CANCER (422-6237)

http://www.cancer.gov

PHARMACEUTICAL ASSISTANCE PROGRAMS

A number of nonprofit organizations offer help with medical expenses such as copayments and deductibles. Eligibility rules may apply. You also may want to contact the drug company that makes your medication to see if a patient-assistance program is available.

Cancer*Care* Co-Payment Assistance Foundation

(866) 55-COPAY (552-6729)

http://cancercarecopay.org

Chronic Disease Fund

(877) 968-7233

http://www.cdfund.org

The Leukemia & Lymphoma Society's Co-Pay Assistance Program

(877) 557-2672

http://www.lls.org/copay

Patient Advocate Foundation Co-Pay Relief Program

(866) 512-3861

http://www.copays.org

Partnership for Prescription Assistance (PPA)

(888) 4-PPA-NOW (477-2669)

http://www.pparx.org

ELDER CARE ASSISTANCE

There are a number of nonprofit organizations and federal programs that provide benefits and assistance for the elderly. Many programs are administered through state governments or community-based agencies and offer services such as transportation, meals, homecare, legal assistance, and caregiver support. You may also want to contact your local Department of Aging, which offers a variety of programs and services for seniors.

AgeNet
(888) 405-4242
http://www.agenet.com

Meals on Wheels Association of America
(703) 548-5558
http://www.mowaa.org

Centers for Medicare and Medicaid Services
(877) 267-2323
http://www.cms.gov

US Administration on Aging's Eldercare Locator
(800) 677-1116
http://www.eldercare.gov

OTHER USEFUL RESOURCES

The following resources can provide helpful information regarding caregiver support, advanced care planning, and end-of-life care.

Aging with Dignity
(888) 5-WISHES (594-7437)
http://www.agingwithdignity.org

Family Caregiver Alliance
> (800) 445-8106
> http://www.caregiver.org

Hospice Foundation of America
> (800) 854-3402
> http://www.hospicefoundation.org

Official Information and Services from the US Government for Senior Citizens
> (800) FED-INFO (333-4636)
> http://www.usa.gov

USA.gov is the US government's official web portal created for the public to get online information about government services and resources, including senior health, Medicare and Medicaid, and caregiver support.

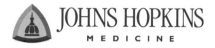

INFORMATION ABOUT JOHNS HOPKINS

The Johns Hopkins Geriatric Oncology Program
The Johns Hopkins Bayview Medical Center
5505 Hopkins Bayview Circle
Baltimore, Maryland 21224

http://www.hopkinsmedicine.org/kimmel_cancer_center/
centers/geriatric_oncology/

The Geriatric Oncology Program brings together practitioners from many disciplines in order to provide a comprehensive approach to the diagnosis, management, and care of older adults with cancer. The program provides a wide range of expert services, including:

- Comprehensive Geriatric Assessment

- Navigation services by a geriatric oncology nurse

- Geriatric psychiatry consultation

- Memory loss and dementia services

- Nutritional support and consultation

- Medication review by an expert pharmacist

- Pain management

- Physical therapy and rehabilitation services

- Palliative care consultation

- Cancer counseling and support groups

- Social work consultation

- Coordination of home care services

- Clinical trials

In the Geriatric Oncology Program, our experts recognize that family members, friends, and your primary medical provider are essential parts of the treatment process. Our consult service and clinical practice are designed to help guide patients and their families through the various options available to them, and to develop a comprehensive plan for successfully coping with the realities of living with cancer.

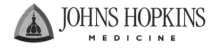

FURTHER READING

Johns Hopkins Patients' Guide to Bladder Cancer, Mark L. Gonzalgo, MD, PhD; Jones & Bartlett Learning, 2011.

Johns Hopkins Patients' Guide to Brain Cancer, Deanna Glass-Macenka, RN, BSN, CNRN; Alessandro Olivi, MD; Jones & Bartlett Learning, 2012.

Johns Hopkins Patients' Guide to Breast Cancer, Lillie D. Shockney, RN, BS, MAS; Jones & Bartlett Learning, 2010.

Johns Hopkins Patients' Guide to Cancer of the Stomach and Esophagus, Mark D. Duncan, MD, FACS; Jones & Bartlett Learning, 2011.

Johns Hopkins Patients' Guide to Cervical Cancer, Colleen C. McCormick, MD; Robert L. Giuntoli, II, MD; Jones & Bartlett Learning, 2011.

Johns Hopkins Patients' Guide to Head and Neck Cancer, Christine G. Gourin, MD, FACS; Jones & Bartlett Learning, 2011.

Johns Hopkins Patients' Guide to Kidney Cancer, Janet R. Walczak, RN, MSN, CRNP; Michael A. Carducci, MD; Jones & Bartlett Learning, 2011.

Johns Hopkins Patients' Guide to Leukemia, Candis Morrison, PhD, CRNP; Charles S. Hesdorffer, MBBCh, MMED; Jones & Bartlett Learning, 2011.

Johns Hopkins Patients' Guide to Lung Cancer, Justin F. Klamerus, MD; Julie R. Brahmer, MD, MSc; David S. Ettinger, MD, FACP, FCCP; Jones & Bartlett Learning, 2011.

Johns Hopkins Patients' Guide to Lymphoma, Aditya Bardia, MD, MPH; Eric J. Seifter, MD, FACP; Jones & Bartlett Learning, 2011.

Johns Hopkins Patients' Guide to Ovarian Cancer, Ritu Salani, MD, MBA; Robert E. Bristow, MD, MBA; Jones & Bartlett Learning, 2011.

Johns Hopkins Patients' Guide to Pancreatic Cancer, Nita Ahuja, MD, FACS; JoAnn Coleman, DNP, MA, ACNP, AOCN; Jones & Bartlett Learning, 2012.

Johns Hopkins Patients' Guide to Prostate Cancer, Arthur L. Burnett, MD, MBA, FACS; Jones & Bartlett Learning, 2011.

Johns Hopkins Patients' Guide to Uterine Cancer, Teresa P. Diaz-Montes, MD, MPH; Jones & Bartlett Learning, 2010.

100 Questions & Answers About Cancer Symptoms and Cancer Treatment Side Effects, Second Edition, Joanne Frankel Kelvin, RN, MSN, AOCN; Leslie Tyson, MS, APRN, BC, OCN; Jones & Bartlett Learning, 2011.

100 Questions & Answers About Caring for Family or Friends with Cancer, Second Edition, Susannah Rose, MS, MSW, PhD; Richard T. Hara, PhD; Jones & Bartlett Learning, 2011.

100 Questions & Answers About Chronic Illness, Robert A. Norman, DO, MPH, MBA; Linda Ruescher; Jones & Bartlett Learning, 2011.

Everything You Need to Know About Cancer in Language You Can Understand, Matthew D. Galsky, MD; Jones & Bartlett Learning, 2010.

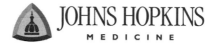

GLOSSARY

Adjuvant therapy: Treatment given after the primary treatment to increase the chances of a cure, and treatment to prevent the cancer from recurring.

Advance Directive (AD): Sometimes known as a living will, this is a written or oral record of what you do or do not want for your health care if you are faced with a life-threatening illness and cannot speak for yourself. An oral AD may be completed when a patient talks with a healthcare provider and a note about the conversation is written into the patient's record.

Anemia: A condition in which the number of red blood cells is too low.

Antiemetics: Antinausea medications.

Biopsy: A procedure in which cells are collected for microscopic examination.

Bone scan: A nuclear medicine imaging study that looks for signs of metastases in the bones.

Brachytherapy: A form of internal radiation therapy.

Cachexia: Physical wasting with loss of weight and muscle mass caused by disease.

Cancer: The presence of malignant cells.

Carcinogen: Cancer-causing substance.

Carcinoma in situ: Very early stage cancer that involves only the place in which it began and has not spread to neighboring or distant tissues.

Carcinomas: Cancers that form in the surface cells of different tissues.

Catheter: A thin, flexible tube inserted into the body to permit introduction or withdrawal of fluids or to keep the passageway open. For example, an intravenous catheter (IV) is inserted into a vein and a urinary catheter is inserted into the bladder through the urethra.

Cells: Basic elements of tissues; the appearance and composition of individual cells are unique to the tissue they compose.

Chemo brain: Difficulty with cognitive functioning as a side effect of receiving chemotherapy.

Chemotherapy: The use of chemical agents (drugs) to systemically treat cancer.

Clinical trial: A large-scale study of a new drug or treatment.

Colectomy: The surgical removal of any extent of large intestine (colon).

Comorbidity: A disease or disorder someone already has prior to a new diagnosis. Examples include diabetes, heart disease, and a previous history of blood clots.

Comprehensive Geriatric Assessment (CGA): A multidimensional, interdisciplinary diagnostic process to assess an older person's medical, psychological, and functional capability. It is used to develop a coordinated and integrated plan for treatment and long-term follow-up.

Cystoscopy: Procedure in which a physician (usually an urologist) uses an instrument to view the inside of the urethra and bladder.

Deconditioning: The deterioration of muscle related to a sedentary lifestyle, debilitating disease and its treatment, or prolonged bed rest.

Drains: A small tube inserted into a wound cavity to collect fluid.

Endoscopy: The use of a flexible scope to evaluate the intestinal tract.

Epstein-Barr virus: A type of herpes virus that causes infectious mononucleosis and can cause lymphocytes to grow abnormally. This virus may cause some types of lymphoma and head and neck cancer.

Estrogen: Female hormone related to child bearing.

Estrogen receptor (ER) positive cancer: Cancer that grows more rapidly with exposure to the hormone estrogen.

Field: The treatment site.

Healthcare proxy: A document that permits a designated person to make decisions regarding your medical treatment when you are unable to do so.

HER2neu overexpression: An excess of the HER2neu protein on the surface of a cell that may be related to a high number of abnormal or defective cells. Herceptin and Tykerb (lapatinib) are targeted therapies used to treat breast cancers that overexpress the HER2neu oncogene.

Hormone receptors: A protein on the surface or inside of a cell that connects to a certain hormone (estrogen or progesterone) and causes changes in the cell.

Hormonal therapy: Treatment that blocks the effects of hormones upon cancers (usually breast and prostate) that depend on hormones to grow (also referred to as endocrine therapy).

Human papillomavirus (HPV): Any of the various strains of papovavirus that causes warts, especially of the hands, feet, and genitals, with some strains believed to be a causative factor in cancer of the cervix, tonsil, and tongue base.

Hypertension: High blood pressure.

Incidence: The number of times a disease occurs within a population of people.

In situ: *See* Carcinoma in situ.

International Prognostic Index (IPI): A system used to determine the prognosis of patients with lymphoma.

Intestinal motility: The spontaneous movement of food and digestive material through the intestinal tract.

Intubation: Tracheal intubation is the insertion of a flexible tube into the windpipe to open and maintain an airway or to allow for mechanical ventilation.

Invasive cancer: Cancer that breaks through normal tissue barriers and invades surrounding areas.

Laminectomy: A surgical procedure done to relieve pressure on the spinal cord or nerve roots. The procedure involves the removal of a portion of the bony arch, known as the lamina, from the back of a vertebra (one of the bones of the spine).

Laparoscopy/laparoscopic surgery: Minimally invasive surgical technique that is performed by inserting an instrument (laparoscope) into the abdomen via small incisions to remove a tumor or the organ containing the tumor.

Lean body mass: All body tissue except storage fat. Lean body mass is made up of structural and functional elements in cells, body water, muscle, bones, and other body organs such as the heart, liver, and kidneys.

Living will: *See* Advance Directive.

Lymph: Fluid carried through the body by the lymphatic system, composed primarily of white blood cells and diluted plasma.

Lymph nodes: Tissues in the lymphatic system that filter lymph fluid and help the immune system fight disease.

Lymphatic system: A collection of vessels with the principle functions of transporting digested fat from the intestine to the bloodstream, removing and destroying toxins from tissues, and resisting the spread of disease throughout the body.

Lymphedema: A condition in which lymph fluid collects in tissues following the removal of or damage to lymph nodes during surgery, causing the limb or area of the body affected to swell.

Malignant: Cancerous; growing rapidly and out of control.

Mastectomy: Surgical removal of a breast to remove a malignant tumor.

Metastasis, metastasize: The spread of cancer to other distant organ sites.

Mini-transplant: *See* Nonmyeloablative transplant.

Mortality: The statistical calculation of death rates due to a specific disease within a population.

Motility: *See* Intestinal motility.

Myelodysplastic syndrome (MDS): Bone marrow disorder in which cells become abnormal and dysfunctional. Some patients with MDS develop acute myeloid leukemia (AML). AML arising from MDS is usually very difficult to treat.

Myeloproliferative syndromes/diseases (MPD): Types of disease marked by the production of excess cells in the bone marrow. MPDs can turn into myelodysplastic syndrome and AML, which can be very difficult to treat.

Myelosuppression: A condition in which bone marrow activity is decreased, resulting in fewer red blood cells, white blood cells, and platelets. It is a side effect of some cancer treatments.

Neoadjuvant therapy: Systemic therapy (chemotherapy or hormonal therapy) or radiation therapy given to people with cancer prior to surgery in hopes of decreasing the size of the primary tumor and preventing the cancer from recurring.

Nephrectomy: Surgical removal of a kidney.

Neuropathy: *See* Peripheral neuropathy.

Neutropenia: A condition of an abnormally low number of a particular type of white blood cell called a neutrophil. White blood cells (leukocytes) are cells in the blood that play an important part in fighting off infection.

Noninvasive cancer: Cancer confined to its tissue point of origin and not found in surrounding tissue.

Nonmyeloablative transplant: Also known as a "mini-transplant," this is a stem cell (bone marrow) transplant that uses lower doses of chemotherapy with or without radiation and immunosuppression that are lower than those used in standard transplants. This method is sometimes used with older patients because the rate of transplant-related complications and mortality is lower than with other approaches.

Oncologist: A cancer specialist who helps determine treatment choices.

Osteopenia: A condition in which bone mineral density or bone mass is less than normal.

Osteoporosis: A condition of abnormal loss of bony mineral density resulting in fragile porous bones and an increased risk for fracture.

Palliative care: Care to relieve the symptoms of cancer and its treatment to maintain the best quality of life.

Pathologist: A specialist trained to distinguish normal from abnormal cells.

Peripheral (sensory) neuropathy: Tingling, numbness, or burning sensations in the hands, feet, or legs caused by damage to peripheral nerves by a tumor, chemotherapy, or radiation.

Phases: A series of steps followed in clinical trials.

Platelets: Blood cells that are involved in clotting and the prevention of bleeding.

Polypharmacy: Polypharmacy means "many drugs" and occurs when a person takes several different medications. Mostly affecting the elderly, polypharmacy is also commonly found in the general population. This can lead to problems including confusion of medicines, doses, or schedule; drug–drug interactions; increased risk of adverse drug reactions; and higher costs for the patient.

Primary care doctor: Regular physician who gives medical check-ups.

Progesterone: A female hormone.

Progesterone receptor (PR) positive cancer: Cancer that grows more rapidly with exposure to the hormone progesterone.

Prognosis: An estimation of the likely outcome of an illness based upon the patient's current status and the available treatments.

Proximal: Toward the beginning, the nearer of two or more items. For example, the proximal end of the arm is the part closest to the shoulder.

Radiation oncologist: A cancer specialist who determines the amount of radiation therapy required.

Radiofrequency ablation: Use of high-frequency alternating current to create frictional heat within the tumor to "burn" the tumor cells to death without the need to actually surgically remove them.

Radiologist: A physician specializing in the treatment of disease using radiation therapy.

Red blood cells: Cells in the blood whose primary function is to carry oxygen to tissues.

Risk factors: Any factors that contribute to an increased possibility of getting cancer.

Stage: A numerical determination of how far the cancer has progressed.

Stent: A tiny tube placed into an artery, blood vessel, esophagus, or other tubular body part (such as one that carries urine or bile) to hold the structure open. Stents are used to palliate symptoms caused by an obstructing tumor mass.

Surgical oncologist: A specialist trained in surgical removal of cancerous tumors.

Systemic treatment: A treatment that affects the whole body (the patient's whole system).

Systolic blood pressure: Blood pressure readings are measured in millimeters of mercury (mmHg) and are given as two numbers (e.g., 120/70). The top number (120) is the systolic blood pressure, which represents the maximum pressure exerted when the heart contracts. The bottom number (70) is the diastolic blood pressure, and it represents the minimum pressure in the arteries when the heart is at rest.

Targeted therapy: Treatment that targets specific molecules involved in carcinogenesis or tumor growth.

Thrombocytopenia: A condition in which the number of platelets is too low. This may result in bruising or serious bleeding.

Tumor: Mass or lump of extra tissue.

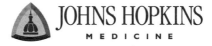

INDEX

friends, support from, 73, 114,
139–140
functional impairment treatment,
117–127
funeral planning, 112–113

gammaknife radiosurgery, 46
gastric cancer, 4–5
gastritis, 5, 87, 97
gastroesophageal reflux disease,
4, 67, 148
gastrointestinal system, 64–66
irritation, 143
G-CSF, 132
geriatric oncologists, 22
geriatric oncology programs, 2, 8,
15–16, 159–160
geriatric syndromes, 27, 66
gingivitis (gum inflammation),
64
Gleevec (imatinib), 54
gliomas, 6
global health, 16, 57, 130
grades of cancer, 5, 12–13
granulopoietic growth factors, 132
guided imagery, 85
gum inflammation (gingivitis), 64
gynecological cancer, 5–6, 49, 52.
See also hormonal therapy

H2-blockers, 145
hair loss, 130
Haldol (haloperidol), 92, 99
Halo braces, 126
hand-foot syndrome, 69
head and neck cancer, 3–4, 124,
148
health care power of attorney
(HPOA), 106–107
health maintenance, 79
healthcare agents, 107
healthcare insurance coverage,
26–28
healthcare proxy, 38, 165

hearing changes, 70–71
heart disease, 61, 131
heart failure, 54
heart risk factors, 51
heartburn, 67. *See also* acid reflux
Helicobacter pylori infection, 4–5
hematological cancers
leukemia, 7, 11, 43, 55, 168
lymphoma, 6–7, 11, 33–34,
43, 55
multiple myeloma, 43, 53, 55
treatment, 49, 53
hepatotoxicity, 51
HER2neu receptors, 3, 54,
165–166
herbs, 137
Herceptin (trastuzumab), 54, 55,
62, 166
high blood pressure (hypertension), 54, 61, 166
high fructose corn syrup, 150
high-calorie protein supplements,
65, 151
Hodgkin's disease, 6–7
holistic care, 117–118
home healthcare services, 138
homeopathic medications, 137
hormonal therapy
adjuvant, 2
androgen deprivation, 52, 135
for breast cancer, 67, 134, 166
for gynecological cancer, 52
for prostate cancer, 52, 135
side effects, 52, 78
systemic therapy, 49
hormone receptors, 3, 52,
165–166, 170
horticultural therapy, 125
hospice care, 96, 99–101, 158
Hospice Foundation of America,
158
human papillomavirus (HPV), 3,
6, 166
hydromorphone, 134